PERSONA AND PERFORMANCE

PERSONA
AND
PERFORMANCE

The Meaning of Role in Drama,
Therapy, and Everyday Life

ROBERT J. LANDY

THE GUILFORD PRESS
New York London

©1993 The Guilford Press
A Division of Guilford Publications, Inc.
72 Spring Street, New York, NY 10012

Printed in the United States of America

This book is printed on acid-free paper.

Last digit is print number: 9 8 7 6 5 4 3 2 1

Library of Congress Cataloging-in-Publication Data

Landy, Robert J.
    Persona and Performance : the meaning of role in drama, therapy,
and everyday life / Robert J. Landy.
      p.   cm.
    Includes bibliographical references and index.
    ISBN 978-0-89862-598-1
    1. Social role.   2. Role playing—Therapeutic use.
3. Psychodrama.   4. Persona (Psychoanalysis)   I. Title.
RC489.P7L35 1993
616.89′1523—dc20   93–2361
                                      CIP

Acknowledgments

Several people have been kind enough to read and critique portions of this book. I am very grateful for the comments and suggestions of Ron Janoff, Robert Taylor, Jim Mirrione, and Irving Wexler. I am especially appreciative of the detailed, thoughtful, and challenging criticism of Eric Miller, Sue O'Doherty, and Alida Gersie. The guidance and advice of Sharon Panulla, Senior Editor at Guilford, was invaluable and I thank her for all her efforts. All of these people's opinions were quite divergent and caused me a good deal of ambivalence. I feel that working it through has made the book considerably stronger.

I also wish to acknowledge my debt to Randi Coen, whose endless hours of research, support, and patience proved invaluable.

I am deeply appreciative of my students at New York University who continue to point me back in the direction of drama therapy even when they are most unsure of what they will find at the end of their journey.

My heartfelt thanks to all those who were willing to reveal their creative, therapeutic process in my presence, believing all the while that drama therapy would make a difference in their lives.

I also wish to acknowledge my debt to a number of thinkers and practitioners within the field of drama therapy—Barbara MacKay, Sue Jennings, Alida Gersie, David Johnson, and Rénee Emunah—who continue to engage me in dialogue compelling enough to restore my faith in the field.

The concepts discussed in Chapter Three were adapted and derived from an article published in the *Journal of the British Association of Dramatherapists*, volume 14, pages 7–15, 1992. Chapter Six of this book is based upon the article, "The Case of Hansel and Gretel," published in *The Arts in Psychotherapy*, Volume 19, pages 231–241, 1992, with permission from Pergamon Press Ltd, Headington Hill Hall, Oxford, UK.

And finally to my family, Katherine, Georgie, and Mackey, who lived through it all—sometimes reading, sometimes eating pages of the manuscript—I say this: My venturing out was a way to make the return that much sweeter.

Contents

A Journeyer
to the Spiritual Mount

Several years ago, I took a sabbatical from my work as an academic. I traveled throughout Britain and Greece, presenting my version of drama therapy to various interested students and mental health professionals. These presentations, however, served as a pretext to get on the trail of ancient, magical places that might touch me in some unfathomable way. I needed distance from the analytical part of myself that all too often informed my daily routines. I wasn't quite sure what I was searching for, but I knew it had something to do with the need to experience transcendence, to feel a new sense of power, and to get closer to an understanding of home by venturing out into the unknown.

In part, I felt like an archaeologist. It wasn't because I collected stones and cultural artifacts from old Druid sites, but because I was in search of more fundamental, less tangible objects—roles. At that point in my thinking, I envisioned roles as archetypes, represented by heroes and fools, victims and survivors—universal forms of thought and action that appear in myths, stories, and dramas. I felt a bit like the sociologist Erving Goffman, who formulated his dramaturgical analysis of social life (Goffman, 1959) by visiting an arcane culture of crofters (subsistence farmers) in the Shetland Islands. Like Goffman, I wanted to know about the ways people present themselves in and out of role; I also wanted to know more about my own presentations in everyday life. So I ventured out to places far away and long ago on a paradoxical journey. My dual purpose was to collect roles and thus learn something about the dramatic nature of existence, and to let go of the need to collect and analyze, opening myself up to the journey.

In the blinding autumn sun in Athens, I inquired about the most

I

extraordinary place I could visit, noting that I was on a spiritual journey. All answered the same: "As a man, go to Mount Athos. But you must be prepared. The experience is very powerful."

Mount Athos is a monastic community on a peninsula in the north of Greece. It is one of the oldest of its kind in the world, and is inhabited by some of the most ascetic men in all Christendom. The spiritual community, like that of the Vatican, has its own government and rules, but it is more severe. Unlike the Vatican, it is far removed from the surrounding urban culture and requires a 2-day journey from Athens by plane, bus, and boat. And unlike the Vatican, it admits only men as pilgrims. Specially trained men carefully scrutinize all arriving visitors to insure that they are indeed of the proper gender.

The inhabitants of Mount Athos are primarily monks, living a nearly medieval existence. A few are more extreme ascetics who reject the communal aspects of the monastery and live a solitary life of devotion; the most radical live in caves chiseled into the lofty mountains, and subsist on offerings left by passing fishermen in baskets hanging down to the sea.

The day before my journey, I was sitting quietly in an Athenian park reading a newspaper when an old Orthodox monk approached, insistently demanding sexual favors. I extricated myself with some effort and wondered, "Was this some sign signifying the dangers of the journey? Was this a trick played by some mythological trickster disguised as a holy man to stir up my sexual and spiritual ambivalences?"

Like all visitors to Mount Athos, I entered not as a tourist but as a pilgrim. I was advised to travel light, for one had to traverse the steep mountains of the peninsula by foot, moving from one monastery to another, a wanderer dependent upon the generosity of the monks for food and shelter. As a pilgrim, I was only allowed to stay at each monastery I visited for one night. The space between monasteries was often vast and the terrain rugged. Occasional huts appeared in between. I stopped at one to ask directions, but quickly exited as my eyes, adjusting to the darkness, focused on a wall lined with skulls. The ancient, massive gates to the monasteries shut tight at sunset. If one was not yet inside, one risked spending the night in the dark woods.

On Mount Athos in September, the sun was brilliantly fierce and the landscape mythical, just as I imagined it had been on Ithaca the day Odysseus returned. An occasional pilgrim passed by with directions toward the next way station, spoken in broken English, French, or German. I understood no Greek at all. All other visible human beings were dressed in black gowns and headpieces, solemn and impenetrable behind their ancient, unshaven faces and leathery skin.

Images of death greeted one everywhere on the mount: the severity of the monks; the bones, fingers, skulls, and other relics of former holy wayfarers, encased behind glass in the chapels; the early morning lamentations performed in crypt-like darkness; the fierce light of the day and eerie silence at night.

There was a companion with me for 2 days. We met on the bus and took the same boat from the small tourist town of Ouronopolis back into time. He was a French actor, dubbed "Alain Delon" by two of the younger monks. I desperately needed him as a companion and helper—one who would ease my fears of the intensity of the light and heat, the Orthodoxy and maleness, the imagery of denial and death. But his presence was disturbing in ways I could not yet fathom. I was aware of his restlessness on the bus. Before we set foot on the boat, he engaged me in a conversation about AIDS. "I am protected," he said. "I will teach you the prayer to protect yourself."

My concerns were already primeval ones—I was about to enter an ancient land that had more to do with the Black Plague. Why was he pushing the terrors of the present upon me?

This Alain Delon flirted glibly with two young monks cleaning squid on the beach in front of our first monastery. They invited us to their cell after curfew, a small crime. In the darkness of their candle-lit domain, the squid cooking in a pot in the outer room, they showed us photographs of young men in civilian clothes; then, abruptly and awkwardly, we made our way back through the dark hallways to our dormitory. Alain, sickened by the fishy odor, had lost interest in them. As for me, I was in a state of suspension, hanging on to every earthy image, yet so out of my element that I could just as well have been in heaven . . . or hell, guided by a French Mephistopheles. Neither Christian nor gay, I found myself standing face to face with my fears of seduction into both forbidden realms.

For the next 24 hours, Alain became a trickster, stirring up as much trouble as he could. He rang the emergency bell outside the dining hall, sending all the monks dashing from their afternoon prayers. He took off his clothes defiantly to swim in the sea near the entrance to the monastery. His antics peaked when with fiendish violence he smashed the spiny body of a sea urchin on a rock facing the chapel, then ridiculed me for refusing to do the same. With each trick, my footing as spiritual searcher seemed to lose hold. I was sinking fast as this presumed helper became my nemesis. The moralist in me condemned his desecration of the holy. "All actors are just philistines, anyway," I thought, "who respect nothing but their own image." I was appalled at this arrogance, which I blamed for steering me away from more righteous reasons for being on this holy mount. I was again on shaky ground—angry and self-righteous, helpless and ashamed.

It was time to part from Alain. I had another 2 days to go. But was I ready to journey alone? Although his presence was humiliating, at least he was familiar. He solved my ambivalence by announcing that he was bored and was going to leave early. Just before heading back to the 20th century, Alain pulled me aside. "Now I will teach you the prayer," he said. "Remember? This will protect you from AIDS, any danger at all. It is very powerful and only known by a few people."

He then proceeded to engage in a series of odd hand movements and uttered a muddled New Age version of the Hail Mary. He wanted me to repeat it. I refused. He did it all again, thinking I wasn't able to follow him. I again refused. He became angry, astonished at my refusal at such a gift. My temper flared, and finding myself sitting on an incipient rage I demanded that he leave. As he left, I heard him laughing, the same demonic laugh he uttered after ringing the bell and watching the frightened men in black rush toward the dining hall. He cursed the monks, and then he cursed me for refusing his offer of grace. In his eyes, I was like them—rigid, self-deceptive, trapped in the oppressive morality and ignorance of the long past. But his final pronouncement was this: "You're just like me, you know . . . even though you are afraid to admit it!"

What did he mean? I stood fearfully alone. Maybe I was like Alain in some ways. Maybe there was a part of me that longed to lash out against all righteous, repressive fathers, despite my rigidity; to open myself up to a feared bisexuality; and to allow myself to believe in prayer and simple protection. It took me a while to calm down. My sense of spirituality and sexuality had been challenged, but I remained intact and ready to move on.

This day was a holiday, the Day of the Cross, and one had to arrive early at a monastery in order to secure a bed. I walked several miles until I approached Simonopetra, carved into the slope of a tall mountain. The path leading up took all my breath away. I was determined to stay the night. A young layperson greeted me and told me that, unfortunately, there was no room. I pleaded, admitting extreme physical and moral fatigue. He took pity on me and assigned me to room with two other Frenchmen.

The first, Jean, on an extended retreat as the spiritual son of a resident monk, was a convert, fully committed to the rules and rituals of Greek Orthodoxy. He was a moralist and intellectual who spoke eloquently of the history and purpose of Mount Athos as a spiritual center and bastion of faith. His friend Jacques, a skeptic, was visiting on the same time frame as myself. His 4 days were about up, and he couldn't wait to return to the sensual shores of the mainland. He missed women most of all and had little interest in the ritual preparations of the monks.

Shortly after a solemn dinner, eaten rapidly as an elder chanted from a holy book, we returned to our cell and the music started. The first waves of the ancient Byzantine chant sent a shock that I experienced in the pit of my stomach. It was the same psychic jolt I had felt days earlier upon my first glimpse of an ancient monastery from the boat spiriting us to Mount Athos. Was this an affliction of all pilgrims, I wondered? Or only those too closed off from their own spirituality?

I followed the sounds into the dark outer room of the chapel. A gathering of pilgrims and monks sat tightly in the orange glow of the inner room. Although afraid to approach, I summoned my moral strength and proceeded, only to be intercepted by Jean, who informed me that only the orthodox were allowed in. My sense of being a pariah, and an angry one at that, surfaced. For that moment, I was the heathen, the Gentile—or, more accurately, the Jew, forbidden to enter the Christian Holy of Holies.

As a pariah, I let the powerful sounds, the smell of the incense, the lush images of half-illuminated icons and precious metal ornaments enter as I stood in my place just outside the door. As if coming out of a trance some 6 hours later, I left the outer room to the few sleeping old monks, and returned to my cell. Jacques was fast asleep, and I attempted to do the same, but the chanting was too intense and my thoughts too insistent. Earlier, at dinner, Jean had hinted that the fathers often displayed their holiest relics on this night, one of which was a piece of the true cross of Christ. Would I miss this while lying in my bed? Would I have been able to see it anyway, in my pariah role, with my Jewish eyes and heart? With these thoughts in mind, I drifted into a sleep of escape. I had seen too much already and could take in no more.

Early the next morning, Jacques and I made the brief, expansive voyage from Mount Athos to Ouronopolis. He informed me matter-of-factly that the holiest relics were rarely displayed. And when they were, they looked quite ordinary. "You missed nothing," he said, "nothing at all."

I took a room with a bath at a good hotel, and we had dinner that night on the *plaka* overlooking the sea. Jacques flirted with an attractive woman who later joined us. In the morning, I caught the bus to Salonika, then a plane back to Athens. Jacques stayed on to pursue a budding relationship.

At every opportunity, like Coleridge's Ancient Mariner at the wedding, I told my story of Mount Athos to a captive listener. The tale was not exactly my albatross, but it has weighed heavily on me. With each telling, I have tried to get closer to making sense of the objective facts of my experience. Over time, that objective reality has faded. The stories told have presented a new reality more akin to fiction. These fictions have served to help me understand some of the roles I encountered on Mount Athos: trickster; helper; orthodox believer; agnostic libertine; chorus of elders, monks, and ascetics; and the central character of myself as hero/searcher, playing out subsidiary roles of coward, victim, angry young man, pariah, witness, and ambivalent one.

As the years pass, the actual models for the characters have assumed a kind of archetypal stature that now belongs to my inner drama. I recognize, for example, the trickster part of me, which on the one hand serves me well when I am stuck in the repressive grip of conventionality and need to ridicule its most orthodox members without undue guilt. But on the other side is the humiliation I fear should my tricks be exposed as crass. Then the trickster role fuels my need to be shamed—a characteristic that has been viewed in current psychological literature as a sense of deep-seated unworthiness (see Lewis, 1971, and Broucek, 1991).

I further recognize parts of myself that function as demon and helper, orthodox and agnostic, intellectual and libertine, coward and warrior. The most powerful role that I recognize is that of the hero/searcher. This role is compelling because it led me to take the journey to Mount Athos in the first place, to stay with the journey, and then to create stories about the journey. As hero, I dare to revise reality in my own way—not as in a psychotic state, marked by a flight from critical thinking, but as in a creative one, where imagination, the ability to invoke meaningful images, reigns. The hero role has taken me through the exercise of writing this book, another battle with the forces of the ascetic fathers. It allows me to enter places I have never been before, or to revisit places as if for the first time. Finally, it allows me to accept the fact that on my heroic journey, I can expect to meet demons of unknown origin.

Mount Athos, an extraordinary place very far away, is just one beginning. All places, even the most ordinary, are arenas in which the psychic struggles of human beings can be played out. For the purposes of this book, those struggles are enacted through role and stories told in role and about roles.

In many ways, this book is a journey. Although it focuses upon the nascent field of drama therapy, it traverses the related landscapes of drama and everyday life. It is my aim to demonstrate how the concept of role serves to connect the three domains, and to provide a role-based model for conceptualizing a healthy personality structure and treating a dysfunctional one.

Role is a basic unit of personality containing specific qualities that provide uniqueness and coherence to that unit. In an earlier paper (Landy, 1990), I have defined role as "the container of all the thoughts and feelings we have about ourselves and others in our social and imaginary worlds" (p. 230). Role as a concept applies to the full range of human experiences through body and sensorium, mind and emotion, intuition and spirit. The concept of role is traditionally a dramatic one, pertaining to the qualities of a specific type of performed character. For many social scientists (see, e.g., Goffman, 1959, and Brissett & Edgley, 1975), role serves as a metaphor useful in analyzing everyday psychological, social, or cultural life in terms of its performance qualities.

For the purposes of this book, I begin with the assumption that the role metaphor linking the world and the stage is a compelling one that has captured the imagination of philosophers, poets, and social scientists at least since antiquity. Burns (1972) points to the continuing use of the metaphor from ancient Greece and Rome (via Plato and Petronius) to the Renaissance (when it was both satirized by Cervantes and elevated to a richly evocative figure of speech by Shakespeare), and well into modern times. The modern world, with few exceptions (see Burke, 1975), turned from the philosophers and poets as interpreters of the *theatricum mundi* to the social scientists. Since the 1930s, these scholars have attempted to revive the notion of world as stage through applying the theatrical metaphor to social life.

I intend to argue, however, that role is more than a powerful metaphor that explains everyday life in terms of dramatic life. As I see it, role is an essential concept that provides coherence to the personality, and that in many ways supersedes the primacy of the concept of self. And by extension, existence is not only played out as in a drama, but is dramatic in its own right. A full understanding of role implies an understanding of the essentially dramatic aspects of everyday existence, which can be highly charged (as in my journey to Mount Athos) or quite ordinary (as in the daily interactions among family members).

Furthermore, I intend to explore the meaning and function of role not only as metaphor and concept, but also as method. The role method will be seen as a means of treating a person in psychological need through drama therapy. For this is a book, after all, about drama therapy—a field that offers an approach to treating social and psychological distress through a role-taking and role-playing process. Throughout the following chapters, I plan to demonstrate how a full understanding of role can provide the field with a solid conceptual base as well as a powerful method of treatment.

In sum, I intend to offer a broad view of role consistent with my understanding of role as the following:

1. A unit of personality.
2. A container of thoughts and feelings.
3. A personality concept.
4. A performed character in theatre.
5. A metaphor for social life.
6. A method of treatment in drama therapy.

Thus conceived, role can serve as a crucial link among drama, everyday life, and therapy. If this is so, then drama therapy, a discipline that attempts to integrate the three domains, may achieve further theoretical clarity through an explication of role.

The book begins with an examination of the origin and development of role both in drama and in the social sciences. An attempt is made to illustrate how role informs personality, and, more generally, how drama informs a world view that is rich in paradox. When the personality conceived of as an aggregate of roles becomes dysfunctional, a form of therapy may be indicated that can redress the disturbances in role. Two clinical case studies are offered—one of an individual, the other of a group—to demonstrate a method of treatment that aims toward restoring a well-functioning role system.

Following the case studies, a system is provided that attempts to categorize the types of roles that seem to recur not only in drama therapy treatment, but also in everyday life. Beginning with a description of everyday role types, I then construct a taxonomy of theatrical roles drawn from repeated types throughout the history of Western dramatic literature. In understanding the nature, function, and style of these roles, I argue, one can better grasp the dramatic nature of healing through role. And in a larger sense, such an understanding can provide dazzled journeyers returning from their own spiritual mounts with a framework within which to make sense of their often contradictory experiences. The book concludes with a discussion of learning to live with role ambivalence, secure in the knowledge that one is indeed complex, willful, creative, and ultimately transformative. A central assumption is woven throughout the book: that well-being depends upon an individual's capacity to manage a complex and often contradictory set of roles.

Throughout, I take a number of liberties within my several roles of storyteller, theorist, and practitioner of drama therapy. I cast my net widely, drawing references and examples from theatre and related arts, the social sciences, popular culture, and personal experience. My discussion of the scholarly literature in these several fields is by no means exhaustive, but rather selective as I build my case for an understanding of role derived from several disciplines, yet based most fully in drama.

The most comprehensive part of my research process concerns a review of some 600 plays in an attempt to extract repeated role types. I am tempted from this part of the process to conclude that role is essentially an unencumbered concept, definable in such simple terms as "the qualities of a character or type in dramatic literature." Yet, in working across disciplines and attempting in part to create a system that addresses psychological dysfunction and everyday existence, I have found that this simple concept transcends its clear boundaries. Given the complexity of role, then, and a chosen method of inquiry that draws upon theoretical, clinical, and anecdotal evidence, this book no doubt ventures out in several directions at once. Ultimately, I intend to return home at the end, this journey done, trusting that the venturing out into the complexities of role is a way to rediscover its simplicity.

CHAPTER ONE

The Origins of Role

HAMLET'S SOLILOQUY
AND THE PARADOX OF DRAMA

Shakespeare's *Hamlet* (1602/1963) begins with a tense scene. A group of soldiers is on guard at Elsinore Castle against the possibility of attack from Norwegian invaders. The soldiers are especially tense because a ghost has appeared to them on two consecutive nights. It is very late and Francisco, about to be relieved of his post for the night, is bitterly cold, tired, and frightened. Barnardo appears suddenly and says: "Who's there?" Francisco responds: "Nay, answer me; stand and unfold yourself."

In its most straightforward meaning, this passage describes two cautious, fearful soldiers asking for each other's identification. However, when Shakespeare writes, "Who's there?", he may be implying more than a question of introduction. The question can be taken as a psychological one: In this dark night of the soul, what part of the psyche is called into being? Neither guard initially recognizes the other; a spiritual darkness is present. Francisco's reply is cautious. He will not divulge his identity until the other agrees to "unfold" himself—an image suggesting a bearing of the psyche, a revealing of secrets.

One psychological reading of Shakespeare's play may be that the entire *dramatis personae* is a reflection of Hamlet, whose inner state may well be projected upon every other character and situation in the play. If Shakespeare's play concerns an unfolding or revealing of the many roles of Hamlet, the first that we see, embodied in the sentinels, is that of the fearful, cautious warrior. As such, Hamlet is guardian of a state in turmoil, on both a political and a psychological level. He is trying to distinguish between one state of being and another: man and ghost, reality and illusion.

The most prominent of Hamlet's roles is that of the ambivalent one. Hamlet is thrust into that role by taking on certain contradictory qualities from his intimates: a murdered father who appears in spirit, a murderous stepfather who proclaims his love, a loving mother who behaves seductively, a lover who is unloving and self-destructive, and friends who are would-be murderers. Hamlet's status as an ambivalent one is most clearly articulated in the most famous of all classical soliloquies, "To be or not to be . . . " Hamlet's musings upon living in a world of knowable causes, or dying into an unknown world of possibly worse effects, come close to the center of the dramatic paradox—a notion that well establishes the connection between the world and the stage, and leads to an understanding of the healing potential of drama.

Paradox is at the heart of the dramatic experience. The individual as actor or group as chorus lives simultaneously in two realities. These realities are diverse: present and past, rehearsal and performance, the studied moment and the spontaneous moment, everyday life and the life of the imagination, internal and external, fiction and nonfiction, the ordinary and the wonderful, the expected moment and the enhanced moment, actor and role, "me" and "not me." Any enactment is dramatic to the extent that it embodies a tension between these or similar states of being. When student actors are exhorted by a teacher, "Stay in the moment," they are also aware that they have rehearsed the scene many times in the past. Past and present meet when one re-enacts a moment "as if" for the first time. In explaining the dramatic paradox of spontaneity and study, we recognize that the spontaneous moment does not appear *ex nihilo*, but is based upon rehearsal.

Perhaps the most significant aspect of the dramatic paradox concerns the notion that the actor and the role are both separate and merged, and that the nonfictional reality of the actor coexists with the fictional reality of the role. This simple dramatic fact, first written about by Diderot (1957), underlies the essential complexity and mystery of the dramatic process, whether applied to everyday life, theatre performance, or therapy.

"En-roling," or entering into a role, implies life; "de-roling" implies death. Yet actors in relationship to roles live, die, and are reborn in new roles over and over again. The actor's dilemma is not to choose between life *or* death, but to find a way to emerge into a state of being that holds life and death together, accepting the inevitable shifts in and out and among several roles. The paradox of drama is to be *and* not to be, simultaneously. Such a task is not a question, as Hamlet's soliloquy would suggest, but an answer.

What, then, is the question? Psychologically speaking, it might be this: How does one cope with difficult contradictions? Or, to link it closer to the plight of the tragic hero, how does one face a terrible truth when one needs desperately to keep it hidden deep within the psyche? The answer is a dramatic one: to be and not to be. Being is the part of the person that is in role, capable of action. Not being is the part of the person that is de-roled, inactive, observing and reflecting upon the acting part. The dramatic paradox is thus a method of survival, in that it allows the actor to act reflectively. It is the stuff of all heroic figures, who dare to search for difficult answers to difficult questions. And it is the stuff of all everyday actors, who dare to act in spite of the often heavy burden of thought and to reflect upon the consequences of their actions.

ROLE AMBIVALENCE

In the following pages, I present a model of understanding human behavior and healing psychological distress through role. At the center of the role model is the notion of paradox, ambivalence, and change. Many roles, by virtue of being played out intensely, indicate their counterparts. The fearful, intellectual Hamlet paves the way for the vengeful man of action. The grounded one searching for a sense of home can be found within the mercurial wanderer. For Odysseus to assert his need to return home to his wife and family, he must take an extraordinary journey into the unknown. Conversely, his wondrous odyssey would have been just another adventure story without the knowledge that the purpose of the going forth is to return and make things right. Each attempt to say, "This is who I am by virtue of the role I play," is easily countered with the thought, "Yes, but what if I were to choose a different role? Wouldn't I also be true to myself?"

In the role of the heroic searcher, I ventured forth into the unknown and thus frightening territory of Mount Athos, as I have described in the Introduction. Yet the coward in me tempered the searcher part. In the paradox of hero–coward, my journey assumed a complexity very different from that of Jacques, the agnostic libertine who became quickly bored with the holy mount and ready to leave on the next boat.

Even in the most extreme commitment to a role, there exists a degree of ambivalence. Try as the ascetics may to push away all thoughts of the flesh, the body still yearns. Even in the meanest cave on the humblest peak of the holy mount, a man full of the holy spirit will drop his basket down to the sea, hoping that a passing fisherman will remember to provide a material form of sustenance. The young monks on Mount Athos took delight in the sexy French actor who reminded them of Alain Delon; the old monk in black, despite his vows of celibacy, demanded sexual favors in an Athenian park; and on the holiest day in the holiest of places, I sat as if before a mirror, with two reflections of myself—Jean and Jacques, the believer and the libertine, contemplating my own struggles of body, soul, and mind.

The ambivalence arising in the clash of body and spirit, of sex and death, presents a primary role conflict that is played out endlessly in the arts, in philosophy, in theology, and in the behaviors of most ordinary people. Hamlet's dilemma of being or not being, of acting or not acting, is truly universal. Most of us do not sit with the overt choice of suicide or parricide, but in dozens of small ways we contemplate little murders and self-punishments for all the ways we have been humiliated by or hurtful to our intimates.

A role does not exist in a singular form. A nurturing mother must also find a way to care for herself. A miser must find a way to spend money or face the fate of King Midas. Hamlet tells us that conscience makes cowards of us all. I would add that the human condition—that of having awareness and the propensity for generating roles—makes us cowards and heroes all at once. To be a coward means to know that there is something important to be afraid of. That knowledge creates the germ of the hero, who, by means of playing out the heroic role, confronts his cowardice and moves on.

Role ambivalence, the clash of feelings engendered in the taking on and playing out of conflicting roles, is the natural order of things. It begins in the tension between nature and nurture—between those role qualities that are inherited, such as appearance, and those that are acquired socially, such as pride or shame based upon one's appearance. And it proceeds as people attempt to build intact, coherent personalities, even though the parts of the personality manifested in thoughts and feelings, desires and needs, often conflict.

Role ambivalence occurs in three ways:

1. Within the role itself when competing qualities conflict, as when, for example, on Mount Athos I tried to play the fearless hero but quickly ran up against my fears along the way.
2. Between two conflicting roles, as when, for example, the fearful quality I experienced manifested itself as the role of coward, which conflicted with the role of hero.

3. As an existential state of being and not being, as when I saw
   myself paradoxically as both hero (not coward) and coward
   (not hero) at the same time.

This third aspect of role ambivalence implies that human beings
can tolerate paradox and negotiate both minor and major conflicts
within and between roles. Even though people tend to seek balance
and order much of the time, that order cannot be realized unless one
is willing to listen to oppositional voices. To seek peace, one must
negotiate with one's tendency to disturb the peace. To do that, one
needs to give voice to one's anger and listen carefully to the message.
In choosing peace, a place needs to be found for war.

This point of view leads to a central assumption of the book:
Although human beings seek balance and integration, they live in
a world of conflicting psychological and social forces that often lead
to imbalance and separation. Many distressed individuals attempt to
avoid uncertainty by limiting conflict and role choice. Shutting out
ambivalence, however, does not necessarily lead to balance, but often
to further distress. By recognizing the ambivalence of being and trying to discover a way to live within and among one's often conflicting roles, one moves closer to a balanced, integrated life.

That balance can be shifted by too little or too much ambivalence. Too little role ambivalence leads to one-dimensional role playing, like that of the workaholic whose identity is inexorably linked
to performance in business. Too much ambivalence leads to confusion
and difficulty with commitment and mastery. At some hypothetical
midpoint, people have the potential to find effective ways to live within and among their roles while accepting the contradictory pulls of
competing personae. Like accomplished jugglers with just the right
number of balls in the air, they move forward, aware that if they take
their precarious state of balance for granted, their balls will tumble
to the ground.

THE ORIGIN OF ROLE IN DRAMA/THEATRE

The juggler is an apt image, as he is a performer, associated with popular forms of performance with roots in the ancient world. Theatre performance is the most prominent source of role, because it is predicated
on the fact that actors take on a mask, persona, part, or character—all
terms synonymous with role—in order to enter into the imaginative
reality of another. Often that other becomes an archetypal figure: a
god or demon, for example, who embodies certain universal quali-

ties. In taking on the role of God, the actor assumes God's primary function—as creator.

Moreno (1960) has pointed to the earliest known usage of the word role (*rotula* in Latin) as a scroll-like object upon which were fastened sheets of parchment, later to be fashioned into volumes used in ancient law courts. In the early theatre of Greece and Rome, the lines of dramatic text were written on the "rolls" and read to the actors by prompters. The character played by the actor came to be known as a role. Yet long before the formal experiments with scripted texts, theatre existed as an expression of the human spirit.

In examining the theatrical sources of role, I offer the premise that throughout the history of theatre, from the early rituals of traditional cultures through contemporary postmodern performances, certain repeated role types have tended to prevail. Evidence of role type is found in ritual, theatre scripts, and other forms of dramatic activity discussed below. A single role, such as the fool, becomes a type when it refers to the universal and generalized qualities of "fool" found repeatedly in dramatic literature and performance. The early gods and demons depicted in ritual activities and ancient forms of theatre in fact have many theatrical counterparts throughout the centuries who have served similar dramatic functions of transformation and transcendence.

A clear source of role is to be found in theatrical scripts or plays, each of which presents a *dramatis personae* or cast of characters. Almost all scripted characters can be conceived as one or several role types. For example, Gertrude, a character in *Hamlet,* can be typed as mother, queen, and lover; Claudius can be typed as father, king, lover, villain, and murderer.

In studying numerous representative plays of Western playwrights from ancient Greece through the present, I have discovered that even though the specific characters change, given changing cultural, stylistic, and historical influences, the role types remain remarkably similar. The heroes and fools, victims and survivors found regularly in Greek and Roman drama are quite prevalent in contemporary American plays and films, for example. Many of these role types are revisited by playwrights because they appear to be archetypal and thus speak to the universal human condition. Dionysus and Medea, Antigone and Orestes are just a few examples.

The notion of repeated role types derived from theatre provides the basis for developing a taxonomy of roles, extracted from the cast of characters of several hundred representative plays spanning recorded history and Western culture. I present the taxonomy later in this book and show how it serves not only as a window into the theatrical origin of roles, but also as a mirror of roles played in everyday life and within the process of drama therapy.

The taxonomy is presented in terms of role type, role qualities, function, and style. By "quality," I mean a measure of the physical, moral, emotional, cognitive, social, and spiritual aspects of the role. "Function" refers to the purpose of particular roles for particular characters, the way roles serve characters as they play them out within the context of their dramatic universe. "Style" refers to the form in which the role is enacted, whether reality-based and representational, abstract and presentational, or somewhere in between. Each style implies a specified degree of affect and cognition—the former implying a greater degree of emotion, the latter a greater degree of cognition.

Although theatre, as represented by plays, is a primary source of role, it is not the only one within the more general sphere of drama. Other dramatic forms include ritual, dramatic play, improvisation, and social drama. Each form embodies some aspects of the dramatic paradox and serves as a source of role.

In its primeval days, more than 5000 years ago, theatre was not about esthetics and commerce, but about worship and mastery of the unknown. The early form of theatre embodied prayer, acts of redemption, and requests for divine intervention, performed by an entire community of celebrants. Select members were often singled out as priests or shamans—those who were practiced in the theatrical art of impersonating the forces of nature and of the gods. The early impersonation involved song and dance, mimesis, the use of masks, and related theatricalized activities.

In taking on and playing out roles such as Rain, the celebrants hoped to insure a productive planting season. In the role of the Warrior God, the celebrants hoped to insure victory in the forthcoming battle. In the role of Death, the celebrants hoped to secure some of the ferocious power reserved only to that deity. Each role enactment seemed to have a specific function. Yet a generalized function emerges from many of the early dramatic rituals—to assert power over that which is inherently more powerful than any human being (e.g., destiny, birth, life, death, afterlife). Through impersonation of nature and the gods, early traditional cultures sought transformation from limitations to boundless power and knowledge, and transcendence from human to divine, from the victim of fate to its master.

The style of the early impersonations was mimetic and presentational, relying on stylized movements and sounds. Early forms of dance, song, and chant, as far as we know, retained an essentially poetic and mythic quality (see Kirby, 1975, and Brockett, 1990). Through their highly stylized, impressionistic art, the early actors played the roles of the visible forces of nature and the invisible forces of the supernatural.

In the religious and cultural rituals of communities, the celebrants commit an act of faith in the present by symbolically re-presenting a story or image from the past. The faith of Christians and Jews, for example, is reasserted in the two symbolic rituals of communion, the Eucharist and Passover. The body of Christ and the aspects of the exodus from Egypt re-emerge in the ritualistic breads and wines consumed in the present. As the celebrants consume the metaphorical sustenance, they take in a bit of the spiritual life—taking on, in some ways, the role of the suffering servant or the exile in the desert. For Roman Catholics and members of the various Orthodox faiths, the drama of Christ's death and resurrection is played out at every Eucharist. The paradoxical meeting of past and present realities is deepened in the belief in transubstantiation, the notion that Christ is actually rather than symbolically present in the bread and wine.

Ritual and religious practices imply a belief in universal forms. As a source of role, these forms essentially recapitulate the function of early theatre, which concerned the transcendence and transformation provided by the gods. In identifying with nature or supernatural sources of power, individuals transcend their limited status as fallible human beings. In ritual, then, one assumes a transcendent role, that of a god or godlike being, in order to assert one's sense of control. Furthermore, in ritual one is part of a meaningful community of celebrants. From that function arises the dramatic role of chorus, the collective voice of the people. Both as transcendent god and earthbound chorus, the individual in worship assumes several key roles.

In dramatic play, characterized as that involving impersonation and/or identification (Courtney, 1974), children symbolically recreate some aspects of their everyday lives through an imaginative process. A doll becomes animated, for example, through the projection of children's feelings. As such, children are simultaneously themselves and another, the doll. Their realities of the everyday and the imaginative are likewise coexistent. The functions of play are multifarious, but for the purposes of this book, children play to make sense of themselves in the world, to master a piece of reality. That mastery occurs as they move in and out of role.

In dramatic play, children generate roles spontaneously and thus unconsciously. If one accepts the premise that play is genetically given (see Huizinga, 1955), then the roles generated in such play would also seem to have a genetic base. As a source of role, dramatic play provides a window through which to view the ways that children and older individuals develop role concepts based in gender (see Grief, 1976), family (see Bruner & Sherwood, 1976), and culture (see Csikszentmihalyi, 1990). In its application to healing, play has become a form of psychotherapy useful for treating children, which proceeds as clients take on roles and play them out in the presence of the therapist. Although the psychoanalytic tradition of play therapy begun by Melanie Klein (1932) views play as a means to an end, that of verbal analysis, alternative traditions based in art and drama therapy view play as both the means and the end of healing (see Landy, 1986).

Improvisational forms of drama involve a spontaneous response to a series of verbal or visual cues. One improvises freely to play, to amuse oneself, or to entertain others. Improvisation is nonscripted and unrehearsed. It is a form of free association, in which the imagination of the actor leads to some unpremeditated form of expression through word, sound, and/or movement. In this case, the dramatic paradox of staying in the moment, of spontaneity, becomes most visible. A present imaginative moment, however, is tempered by a past life of the imagination. The great wits and improvisers, such as Groucho Marx and Robin Williams, often improvise around well-rehearsed themes that have been developed over many years.

Improvisation is in many ways a form of adult play. Thus, as a source of role, it too generates the role of player—one who attempts to master reality through playing in the realm of the fictional. Improvisational activity implies that roles are not simply given to the players at birth, but also generated by the players. Improvisers are creative beings whose greatest creation, perpetually in the making, is their own identity.

In the heightened moments of conflict and tension within a community, the antagonists move into a dramatic mode and engage in a kind of social drama (see Turner, 1982) that carries the potential of either reaffirming or altering the structures and events of everyday life. Suddenly, during a challenge to the social order (e.g., the bombing of Pearl Harbor), the ordinary and the expected are turned around. The social drama carries with it not only the dramatic paradox of two realities, but the potential for transformation and even cataclysm.

Social drama becomes a source of role as an individual or community is challenged by a threat from the outside. Within the social drama one is given the opportunity to stretch beyond one's expected parameters. In this sense, the new possibilities of being arise from the environment. One does not necessarily choose to become a soldier, but is thrust into that role during wartime. In the social drama that arises in Elsinore Castle, Hamlet, the intellectual, is thrust into the role of warrior and killer. It may be that such roles reside within each person's psyche. But it often requires an external event, a social drama, to prod that role potential into being.

THE ORIGIN OF ROLE IN THE SOCIAL SCIENCES

Until the 1930s, with some notable exceptions (see, e.g., James, 1890/1950, and Cooley, 1922), role remained a term fully associated with dramatic activity. With the proliferation of social science research during and since the 1930s, role became a metaphor applied to psychological and social analysis. Finally the poetic notion of world as stage had achieved scientific respectability. Anthropologists, sociologists, and social psychologists began to redefine role in terms of their own theatre of operations—the tribe, the family, the community, the society, and (for the generals) the battlefield. But before they analyzed behavior and culture through the lens of role, they needed to wrestle with the larger concept of self—the source from which, in the opinion of many, all roles flow.

Defining the Self

Early in *Hamlet,* Laertes is about to embark on a trip abroad to seek his fortune. His father, Polonius, the foppish lord Chamberlain, offers well-intentioned parental advice, the most famous of which is this (Act I, scene iii, 78–80):

> This above all: to thine own self be true.
> And it must follow, as the night the day,
> Thou canst not then be false to any man.

Long before Shakespeare's day and long after, philosophers, poets, and theologians professed the idea of a core self that contains the essence of one's being and that can be known. Polonius's version of the Socratic dictum "Know thyself" sums up much classical and modern thinking about the self. It is a thing of permanence that is sometimes at odds with other parts of the person, most notably the false parts that some would call "subselves," "roles," or "social masks." If we can know how to access the true self, they would argue, then we can circumvent the power of these false parts. Implicit here is a moral notion—existence as a struggle between the authentic and God-given forces of light, and the inauthentic and demonic forces of darkness.

In the 1950s and 1960s, the psychologist Carl Rogers (1961) offered a phenomenological theory of personality based on the notion of a primary self as whole and good. Like his contemporary Abraham Maslow (1962), he viewed psychological life as a movement toward self-actualization, a tendency to develop a functional and healthy state of being. His seminal work touched off a movement of humanistic psychologists, many of whom were influenced by Eastern philosophies and aimed, in part, toward uncovering the primary self. This point of view was optimistic and positive, in stark contrast to that of the earlier European psychologists schooled in the analytical approaches of Freud and Jung, who conceived of the self as a battlefield between the forces of id and superego, death and life instincts, shadow and godly archetypes.

Polonius would agree with the notion of self proclaimed by the humanistic psychologists, as would many spiritual thinkers of both East and West, who conceptualized the essential nature of the human being as godlike. Many social scientists, however, began to see the self as broken down into components. According to G. H. Mead (1934) and William James (1890), among others, the self is comprised of an "I" and a "me." The "I" is an objective, generalized set of permanent attributes, and the "me" is a subjective, more specific set of behaviors determined largely by social circumstances. Moreover, as Mead put it, "We divide ourselves up in all sorts of different selves with reference to our acquaintances. . . . There are all sorts of different selves answering to all sorts of different social reactions" (1934, p. 142). James out it similarly: " . . . a man has as many social selves as there are individuals who recognize him and carry an image of him in their mind" (1890, Vol. 1, p. 294).

Thus self becomes a social construct, and human beings build their identities on the basis of the ways they are seen by others. To carry images of others means to see them and to act toward them in certain prescribed ways. If I see my daughter as independent and strong, and act toward her as if she possessed these traits, then she will conceive of herself as independent and strong. If her teachers see her as dependent and helpless, then she may also incorporate that contradictory self-image. In fact, to use Charles Cooley's (1922) image of the "looking-glass self," each person or group that we encounter reflects back a sense of who we are.

Such a multifarious conception of self naturally implies certain splits or contradictions within the person. James stated:

> From this there results what practically is a division of the man into several selves; and this may be a discordant splitting, as where one is afraid to let one set of his acquaintances know him as he is elsewhere; or it

may be a perfectly harmonious division of labor, as where one tender
to his children is stern to the soldiers or prisoners under his control.
(1890, Vol. 1, p. 294)

It is in these splits that human beings discover their humanity. The
harmonious ones lead them to engage in their contradictory roles
with energy and challenge; the discordant ones lead to anxiety, shame,
and fear, the darker sides of the psyche.

The notion of the self shared by James and the group of social-
psychological theorists known as the symbolic interactionists is close
to my understanding of role as multifaceted, derived in part from the
social world, and essential in building the human personality. Yet this
notion contradicts the sense of self as true, good, and indivisible.
Despite the moral weight of many theologians, philosophers, poets,
and humanistic psychologists, the concept of self as monolithic,
monotheistic, and authentic oversimplifies human existence. This
conception implies that the aim of existence is to get back to the core
being, the innocence and perfection of the child, the oneness of God,
the goodness of the self. To do so, one must struggle through all the
false selves, the dark, inauthentic roles that block the way. This myth
of the self is certainly seductive, especially during times when one
recognizes one's helplessness in the face of addiction, abuse, war,
or poverty. It then becomes heartening to know that there is a
deeper good, a central intelligence that with great effort can be accessed. In religious practices, that core self is linked with God, well
expressed in the notion that the kingdom of God is within each
person.

Yet when one fully indulges in this idea of self, one may, like Nar-
cissus, drown in one's own monolithic image. In the beginning of
life, when one's experience is limited to that which one takes in
through the senses, a strong argument can be made for a monoself,
a core being that is whole and good. But as one develops consciousness and social relationships, that core begins to lose its purpose,
which is to support a life that is new and undeveloped. Perhaps it
remains as a vestigial organ, an artifact, a reminder that once upon
a time we were unencumbered and innocent.

In a nuclear age, all things once considered indivisible are now
splittable. Not only have we split the atom, but also families through
divorce and abandonment, communities through racial segregation,
nations through holy and civil wars, cultures through assimilation,
and the self. In splitting the self, one enters a new mythological
system—one that is not only polytheistic, but also, paradoxical. In a
postnuclear age, the maxim "God is dead" is a cliche. A more appropri-

ate motto for our purposes would be "The self is dead," at least in its monolithic version.

In the new mythology there is a need for stories that support the multitude of splits confronted each day on personal and political levels, well exemplified by the scourge of AIDS, which leads to the breakdown of both the immune system and the community. And there is a need for stories that address the consequences of these splits as we confront issues of power and status, intimacy, bearing and raising children, searching for meaningful vocational and leisure activity, dying, and burying the dead. These stories need to be peopled not with a self, but with roles that respond to the many ambiguities of being.

The poet William Butler Yeats (1921/1956) well characterized the modern era as one where "Things fall apart; the centre cannot hold." If God is dead and the self is dead, why require a center? Peel away the layers of the onion and nothing is there. In a culture of multiple choices, one needs a way to think about or play out the different parts. One way is through role. And as we shall see later, when role becomes a concept in its own right, that concept is not so glib that it denies the existence of all that God and self once represented and still represents to many.

From Self to Role

James and Mead had a timely idea in conceiving of the self as dual and multiple. They merely used an imprecise term, as "self" is too easily limited to the fixed moral entity of Polonius via Shakespeare. The term role is more apt, as it addresses the dramatic and paradoxical nature of existence.

Mead was actually the first among social scientists to employ the role metaphor, although role remained in the service of the self. Mead used the term role taking to specify the social and symbolic development of the mind and the self. He stated:

> It is generally recognized that the specifically social expressions of intelligence, or the exercise of what is often called "social intelligence," depend upon the given individual's ability to take the roles of, or "put himself in the place of," the other individuals implicated with him in given social situations; and upon his consequent sensitivity to their attitudes toward himself and toward one another. (1934, p. 141)

Linton (1936) defined role as a collection of rights and duties ascribed to a social status. For Linton, role is socially determined but also behaviorally oriented, propelling a person of a particular status into action. Linton conceived of two kinds of roles, roughly equivalent to James' I and me: the first, a general objective role incorporating all other roles and determining one's social status; and the second, specific, more subjective roles based in those rights and duties that one acquires from the social world.

Neither Mead nor Linton actually viewed role as a viable concept in its own right. To them it was a social artifact subsidiary to the more inclusive concept of self. As Mead saw it, the trinity of mind, self, and society determines human behavior. For the early social scientists, then, role was merely a serviceable metaphor.

The founder of psychodrama and sociodrama, J. L. Moreno, conceived of his therapeutic and epistemological system as based in an understanding of human beings as role players. Moreno was openly critical of Mead and Linton for limiting role to a social source. As Moreno (1960) saw it, role has three primary dimensions: the psychosomatic, pertaining to such basic body functions as eating and sleeping; the psychodramatic, pertaining to fantasy and inner psychological processes; and the social, pertaining to relationships in the social world. The first two aspects, concerning physically and psychologically based roles, precede the development of social roles.

Moreno, a scion of early 20th-century Vienna, was trained medically as a psychiatrist but found the clinical approach to treating mental illness too constricting. He then looked to his other passion, theatre, as a more creative methodology for healing. But Moreno quickly rejected what he saw as the conservative trend toward producing old and tired plays. He turned instead to the more open approach of improvisation, fueled by the spontaneous presentation of self through role. In fact, he began an early form of improvisational and political theatre in Vienna (see *The Theatre of Spontaneity,* Moreno, 1947). Yet within a few years his work moved away from the theatre. In time, his language began to resemble the social scientists' understanding of the dual nature of self located in the social world. In describing the form and function of role, for example, Moreno (in Fox, 1987) wrote: "The form [of role] is created by past experiences and the cultural patterns of the society in which the individual lives" (p. 62); "The function of the role is to enter the unconscious from the social world and bring shape and order to it" (p. 63). Echoing the notion of "I" and "me," he stated (in Fox, 1987): "Every role is a fusion of private and collective elements. Every role has two sides, a private and a collective side" (p. 62).

Yet Moreno took a giant step beyond Mead and his colleagues in conceiving of the human being as a role player, rather than simply a role taker. Mead's theory is a cognitive one. Role is part of self, which is immersed in mind. Like the Cartesian notion of *Cogito, ergo sum*, Mead's sense is that cognition precedes existence—or, more precisely, that cognition in concert with social factors determines the shape of the self: I think and I interact; therefore I am.

Moreno's theory of role is an active and interactive one. The personality is developed as one plays out the many possibilities of being. These possibilities include playing real or ideal roles of protagonist, auxiliary ego, double, and director. The protagonist is the central figure in the psychodrama. Auxiliary egos are antagonists, or those who challenge or support the protagonist. The double is an alter ego, representing the inner thoughts and feelings of the protagonist and auxiliary egos. And the director is the leader of the psychodrama, who moves the other players in and out of role and generally attempts to explore and resolve a protagonist's dilemma.

Moreno is also credited with developing a social form of psychodrama, which he called "sociodrama." Within this form small groups of individuals examine tangible social issues, such as racism and sexism, through taking on somewhat abstract adversarial social roles and engaging in a directed encounter. A group may, for example, dramatize issues of race through the identification of antagonists and the taking on and playing out of an improvised scenario between those groups identified. The attitudes dramatized may well cause tension within those who deny their identification with the racist role; in living through the dramatic paradox of "me" and "not me," such attitudes can be uncovered and worked through. The sociodramatic form points to the notion that roles are culturally and socially determined. Through the therapeutic process of sociodrama, one is able to examine one's tendency to stereotype and defame groups of people, or oneself as representative of that group.

Even if he did not break with all the reigning theories he critiqued, Moreno offered a viable system of social analysis and therapy based in role. In his system, the capacity to generate roles spontaneously appears to be given at birth, even as it is subject to environmental and social influences.

In his classic study of social life as drama, *The Presentation of Self in Everyday Life*, Goffman (1959) offered an understanding of role similar to the definition given by Linton over 20 years earlier. As Goffman defined it, role is "the enactment of rights and duties attached to a given status" (p. 16). Yet he went beyond the cognitive and social notions of self. Self—and, by implication, role (he tended to equate the two)—is "a dramatic effect arising diffusely from a scene that is presented" (p. 253). Within Goffman's world view, life is theatrical and identity is a presentation of ourselves in role to a particular audience.

At the end of his study, Goffman denuded the dramatic metaphor. Although life is dramatic, there are further metaphors to mine regarding the nature of social life. For Goffman in 1959, role was a handy allusion, useful for analyzing societies but not compelling enough to lead to a more fully developed role theory.

Theodore Sarbin is the social psychologist who has worked most directly with the concept of role, extending it into a new discipline, that of narrative psychology. Like his predecessors, Sarbin sees role as socially determined, but he moves beyond them in his concise conceptualization of role as "a patterned sequence of learned actions or deeds performed by a person in an interaction situation" (1954, p. 225). He also moves ahead in his extensive focus upon the dimensions of what he terms "role enactment," a process that concerns number of roles, organismic involvement, and pre-emptiveness or time.

For Sarbin, the functional person is one who can play a wide variety of roles—those that appropriately correspond to a variety of social circumstances. The quantity of roles one plays is significant in the sense that one has many options, many faces and facets.

"Organismic involvement" refers to the style of one's role enactment, the degree of affect or intensity one gives to a role. Sarbin (Sarbin & Allen, 1968) conceives of a continuum that begins with noninvolvement and proceeds to casual role enactment, ritual acting, engrossed acting, classical hypnotic role taking, histrionic neurosis, ecstasy, and sorcery and witchcraft. Sarbin's model thus takes into consideration not only the ways in which we play out our ordinary roles, but also those extraordinary states found in worship, sex, mental illness, and trance. His continuum is similar to the distancing model that I have adapted from Scheff (1979) (Landy, 1983, 1986) to conceptualize, in part, drama therapy. It too posits levels of affective involvement in the playing of a role, limiting the points on the continuum to three:

1. "Overdistance," similar to Sarbin's noninvolvement, is characterized by a minimal degree of affect and a high degree of rational thought that removes one from one's own feelings and those of others.

2. "Underdistance," similar to histrionic neurosis, is marked by an overabundance of feeling that floods one's objectivity and reflective capacities.

3. "Aesthetic distance," similar to engrossed acting, is notable for a balance of affect and cognition, wherein both feeling and reflection are available.

The dimension of "time" in Sarbin's model is a comparative one, referring to the amount of time one spends in playing out, for example, a work role in relation to the time spent in playing, for example, a domestic role.

In a further development of his ideas, Sarbin (1986) has extended role into story. Role players become storytellers who make sense of their existence through framing a narrative about their lives in role. The focus of analysis, then, is on the dual roles of protaganist within one's story and teller of one's story, similar to those of actor and observer or participant and observer, or James's and Mead's "I" and "me." With this direction, Sarbin has fully embraced drama as the primary frame of reference for an analysis of social life: As people take on and play out roles based in the events that make up their lives, they frame stories about themselves in role, which provide an understanding and give meaning to their existence.

Other contemporary psychologists and critics of society and culture, among them Hillman (1983), Bruner (1987), Sacks (1987), and Postman (1992), have subscribed to the notion of life as story and people as characters within their invented life narratives. This point of view reflects the continuing application of the dramatic metaphor in general, and of story and role in particular, to an understanding of social and psychological life. As Postman (1984) suggests, the social scientist may not be a scientist at all, but rather a moral philosopher more concerned with meaningful narrative than with replicable experimentation. With this in mind, let us look at selected examples in the arts of those whose words and images offer further insight into role origins.

SELECTED EXAMPLES OF ROLE IN LITERATURE AND VISUAL ART

The artist, perhaps more than the social scientist, has responded powerfully to the modern and postmodern concept of multiple selves. Emblematic of the split psyche are the characters of Dr. Frankenstein and his monster, and of Dr. Jekyll and Mr. Hyde in Mary Shelley's (1818/1983) and Robert Louis Stevenson's (1886/1986) respective 19th-century novels.

One of the innovators of the modern psychological novel, Joseph Conrad, created a more complex split between the rational and irrational parts of the psyche. His story "The Secret Sharer," for example, describes two loners, a young sea captain and a fugitive whom the captain secretly stows away in his cabin. In becoming merged with his alter ego, the captain reflects:

He was not a bit like me, really; yet, as we stood leaning over my bed place, whispering side by side, with our dark heads together and our backs to the door, anybody bold enough to open it stealthily would have been treated to the uncanny sight of a double captain busy talking in whispers with his other self. (1912/1964, pp. 30–31)

The romantic Edgar Allan Poe also played with the notion of the double, the alter ego that represents the dark, irrational part of the psyche. In his story "William Wilson," (1839/1966), a young man is plagued by another who bears the same name and same appearance as he. In finally murdering this person, he kills a persona, the irrational part of himself that he could neither embrace nor repress. In killing the double, however, he too dies, a victim of his inability to live in his role ambivalence.

Thus we see again how a notion of self is split, in Moreno's terms, into the protagonist and the double. Literature of the 19th and early 20th centuries is rich in examples of reflections, like that of Oscar Wilde's (1891/1974) *The Picture of Dorian Gray*, and alter egos, like that of Dostoyevsky's (1846/1972) *The Double*.

In contemporary literature and art, we see a further fractionalization of the self into its roles. This is evident in Philip Roth's creation of a fictional double, Nathan Zuckerman, who seems to represent his own autobiographical struggles. In *The Counterlife* (1986), Roth's alter ego offers a direct statement on the demise of the personal self and the rise of the persona. Zuckerman notes that even if there is an "irreducible self" (p. 319), it must be very small indeed, reflecting an "innate capacity to impersonate" (p. 319) rather than a core being. Zuckerman then affirms categorically that he has no self at all, but rather an internal collection of roles, "a troupe of players that I have internalized" (p. 320). And finally, Zuckerman, via Roth, expounds: "I am a theatre and nothing more than a theatre" (p. 321).*

The notion of an internalized, permanent company of actors that comprises one's identity takes concrete form in the tradition of self-portraiture. Each painting is a depiction of a single role or a conglomerate of several related ones. Modern painters have especially taken great liberties in presenting fragmentations of their identities. The early 20th-century Mexican painter Frida Kahlo is a good example, as she depicted intimate aspects of her spirituality, physical disabilities, sexuality, and passionate connection to Diego Rivera through her almost obsessive self-portraits (see Zamora, 1987). These images

---

*In a later offering, *Operation Shylock* (1993), Roth presents a further exploration of the fractionalized theatrical identity by offering up two fictional Philip Roths, one an American-Jewish novelist, the other, a fanatical imposter stirring up trouble in Israel.

of herself are all presented in role, as if Kahlo were costumed for a play about the particular aspect depicted—for example, "Ugly," "Hairless," or "Diego on My Mind," all titles of her self-portraits.

A little-known contemporary of Kahlo, Claude Cahun, a female surrealist, used paint and photomontage in self-portraits to express a fractured conception of sexual and psychological identity. In her critique of Cahun's work, Therese Lichtenstein (1992) writes:

> . . . she is exploring a notion of the self as an accumulation of selves, or a shifting set of social relations, establishing a destabilized self-portrait that posits identity as contingent and mutable. The sense of multiple selves, of masquerade, of gender as a series of conventions . . . prefigures Cindy Sherman's photography . . . which stages stereotypical and historical feminine identities as self-portraits. (p. 65)

Cindy Sherman, a postmodern photographer, well expresses the concept of multiple identity in her self-portraits (see Sherman, 1987). Sherman fully portrays herself as movie star, pin-up, housewife, and other roles associated with media-generated personae of the recent past, lending further testimony to Roth's credo of the individual as a theatre.

For Kahlo, Cahun, and Sherman, role originates both in society and in universal archetypes embedded in the psyche and the culture. The work of these artists reflects the feminist position linking the personal and the political, as their imagery swings from such personal sources as Kahlo's abortions to such cultural ones as Sherman's understanding of media-generated conceptions of women.

Contemporary theatre, video, and film artists have likewise underscored the rise of the multiplicitous role. This can be seen in performances that appear to be peopled by an entire cast of characters, yet are in fact played by one actor moving in and out of multiple personae. Examples of such actors include Lily Tomlin, Whoopi Goldberg, Jeff Weiss, John Belushi, Andy Kaufman, and Eric Begosian. This form of performance art tends to be disturbing in the way that a ventriloquist and a dummy can disturb one's notion of singularity and humanity. One asks: Is there one or many? Who is the real one, and where am I (as onlooker) in relation to this chameleon-like figure?

The filmmaker Ingmar Bergman offers a very different sense of the fractured self, one that is measured and reflective. His use of role is well illustrated in *Persona*, a seminal film demonstrating that the center cannot and should not hold. It concerns a relationship between two differing personality types: a famous, accomplished actress who is suffering a form of acute depression and suddenly becomes mute, and a loquacious, somewhat boorish nurse who is her companion on an isolated island. In juxtaposing the portrait of one upon the other and taking the two through a role reversal, Bergman obliquely comments upon the interchangeable nature of existence. In this provocative film he questions the structure of personality, and rather than offering a direct answer, he hints at its paradoxical and dramatic nature.

Bergman has served as a model for many aspiring art film directors, including Woody Allen. Allen's film *Zelig* provides a further variation on the theme of multiple roles. Zelig is a character whose psychological problem is his propensity for assuming other personae. Allen mines this dilemma for all its comic gold as Zelig—basically an Everyman character, an ordinary *schlemiel*—takes on powerful roles by virtue of associating with the most prominent men of the 1930s and 1940s. Even though Allen's central character, based largely on himself, is consistent from film to film as the fool, the loser, the pariah, and the hypochondriac, in Zelig he has significantly expanded the notion of a core self into that of the polypersonality whose disorder is, in many ways, a condition of normality within a society that demands multiplicity.

Zelig's disorder is very different from clinical multiple personality disorder. Multiple personality is a fairly rare, though much researched, psychological disorder based primarily in severe childhood abuse (see, e.g., Allison & Schwarz, 1980, and Putnam, 1989). The victims defend against the horrors of memory by constructing several alter egos who protect them from the trauma. Both film and video artists have chosen the multiple personality as a topic for exploration. We find fictionalized versions of the multiple personality in such films as *The Three Faces of Eve* and *Sybil*. A television documentary (CBS-TV's *48 Hours*, "The Many Faces of Marsha," February 27, 1991) featured the treatment of one woman in her 40s who manifested more than 200 personalities. Furthermore, the clinical psychologist Richard Noll (1989) has claimed that many of the alter personalities found in individuals with multiple personality disorder correspond to the archetypes identified by Jung in his studies of the collective unconscious.

In multiple personality disorder, role springs from a psychopathological source and becomes a defense against re-experiencing the pain and shame of abusive social relationships. An artist's interest in healthy or pathological roles springs, however, from a conception of the personality as comprising a multitude of roles. In a modern and postmodern sense, the normal personality is assumed to be fragmented as a reality of contemporary life, and the artist's task is to reveal the parts by creating appropriate metaphorical stages upon which they may be played out.

FROM ROLE METAPHOR TO ROLE CONCEPT

Drama, social science, and modern and contemporary art reflect a shift away from a concept of a monolithic self. In the absence of a self, however, many will still need to look to a notion of a central intelligence that frames the personality. If at the core of the human personality is not a thing, a godlike self, perhaps we can conceptualize a dramatic process—that of impersonation, the ability of the developing person to fashion a personality through taking on and playing out various personae or roles.

Consistent with the idea of the multitudinous personality, role can be seen as a concept in its own right as it relates to a larger model of personality and healing. In moving beyond the *theatricum mundi* metaphor, the concept of role implies not only that the world is a stage and the people are players, but that the space between reality and imagination is the source of creative energy enabling us to make sense of our perhaps not-so-meager existences. By being simultaneously actors and characters, ordinary human beings and something else—gods, demons, heroes, villains—we are capable of transforming our understanding, feeling, and valuing. These transformations are at the heart of the dramatic role-taking and role-playing process, whether in drama, therapy, or everyday life.

As people develop and in essence reveal their *dramatis personae*—a cast of characters who are able to contain and express their complex thoughts, feelings, and values—they fashion a rich and full personality, which I conceive as a system of interrelated roles. Yet being a multiplicity of things can cause role ambivalence. When roles retreat into isolation or do battle with one another or join together in an unholy alliance to fight a common external enemy, a person experiences distress that can run the gamut from mild anxiety to severe emotional disturbance.

Drama therapy can be very useful in working through such distress as it proceeds through role. In drama therapy, both client and therapist move in and out of fictional roles in order to lay claim to the best-functioning everyday ones. Protagonists generally do not enact scenes from their actual lives; instead, they project aspects of themselves onto an object or fictional role, such as a puppet, a character in a story, or a miniature figure in a sandbox. The heart of the dramatic paradox of actor and role, of "me" and "not me," becomes most clearly visible in this form of dramatic healing. Although clients work in role, the process also encompasses a movement out of role, as they reflect upon their enactment and attempt to extract its meaning. Ultimately, the drama therapy client seeks to construct an internal system of roles that translates into meaningful action in the world.

In drama therapy, role is the form of one's dramatic action. The content of that action is embodied in stories. The story is the container of one's roles. It is told from a single point or from multiple points of view, each one representing a role. Later, in the case of Hansel and Gretel (see Chapter Six), I describe an example of group drama therapy, in which each member of the group is asked to retell the story from the point of view of a chosen character. In this case, several versions of the story were told in the roles of Hansel, Gretel, the Mother, the Gingerbread House, and so on. Each story told in role represents an individual storyteller's psychological and aesthetic point of view. And each story presents at least two roles—that of the storyteller, and that of the subject of the story.

Story, then, is a form of drama that examines, among other things, the often paradoxical relationship between the narrator and the characters and events narrated. Like other forms of dramatic activity, it exists between the two realities of the fictional and the non-fictional, for each true story that people tell about their lives becomes a version of that truth and thus a part-fiction in the telling. Conversely, even the most outrageous fiction, once committed to story form, contains some grain of truth as it relates in some basic way to the imagination of the storyteller.

The role as seen in drama therapy is the container of one's dramatic action. It is a form, an expression in behavior containing feelings, thoughts, and values associated with a single persona, rather than with a total personality. It is part rather than whole, a single point of view among others. Without role, there can be no story. A role can exist without a story, but requires a story in order to communicate its essence.

In its inderdisciplinary nature, drama therapy offers an eclectic and inclusive notion of role as a concept in its own right. Taking a broad view of role origins allows drama therapists to conceive of role as genetically based, as in play; archetypal, as in theatre; and subject to influence by culture, environment, and social interaction.

The final shift of role from metaphor and concept to therapeutic method is discussed in Chapter Three. But first, I turn to a discussion of how the concept of role relates to the psychological development of human beings.

CHAPTER TWO

The Development of Role

Role as a concept derived from drama and the social sciences, and reflected in the arts, may well serve as a cornerstone for conceptualizing personality structure and psychological healing through drama therapy. If so, it is essential to discuss the ways that roles develop in the life of a human being. In this discussion, it is assumed that roles are influenced by genetic as well as by environmental and cultural factors. It is further assumed that although roles are expressed behaviorally, they also include cognitive, affective, social, and spiritual aspects. To acquire roles, the human being becomes role recipient, role taker, and role player.

THE HUMAN BEING AS ROLE RECIPIENT

The earliest roles, those pertaining to the simple biological needs of the organism, appear *in utero*. The developing fetus satisfies its somatic needs through assuming the roles of breather, sucker, eater, expeller, sleeper, and mover. These roles are automatically played out by the fetus. These and related somatic roles are primary roles, in that they are given genetically and are essential to the survival of the fetus.

At birth, the infant asserts all these roles in order to survive in a less protected environment. Soon a new role surfaces—that of the interactive social being, who needs to be touched and held by the parents or caregivers in order to continue to develop. Furthermore, the primary uterine roles expand to accommodate to both the new environment and the new people responsible for providing food, comfort, and protection. Infants receive these primary roles as a birthright.

They are given, unlearned, inherited. The quality of the roles—that is, how infants play out their roles of breather, sucker, eater, expeller, sleeper, mover, and interactor—is based in certain genetic predispositions further influenced by the social, physical, and psychological environment. These factors determine such qualities as the strength or weakness of the sucking instinct; the length and depth of sleep; and pleasure or resistance associated with feeding, defecating, moving, and hugging.

Primary somatic roles function to perpetuate the individual's existence. Notable exceptions include roles of gender and ethnicity, which do not relate to one's struggle to survive, at least on a biological level.

In normal development, the somatic roles work in harmony with one another; for example, the role of eater supports those of breather, sucker, mover, and defecator. Outside the womb, eating becomes a social act and therefore requires a relationship with a feeder. At first holding the infant to feed, then simply holding the infant to satisfy its needs to be held, the parents contribute to a healthy interactive role development.

In abnormal development, the role system, an internal structure that holds individual roles in relationship to one another, becomes imbalanced for a number of physiological and psychological reasons. A single role may be underdeveloped because of a genetic predisposition or physical illness. An obstruction in the lungs or bowels, for example, affects the role of breather or defecator. A problem with any one primary role will influence the rest of the role system. Difficulty in breathing, for example, may affect the way an infant plays out the roles of sucker, eater, and mover. With appropriate assistance from caregivers, the infant can learn both to strengthen the underdeveloped role and to utilize the more fully developed ones as a means of compensation. With insufficient environmental support, a poorly developed somatic role may weaken further, and thus affect the rest of the system negatively.

Furthermore, if a single physiologically healthy role is denied appropriate environmental support, it too may adversely affect the role system. For example, the interactive role of one who is held and nurtured may be diminished by virtue of the negligence of the primary caretaker. As a consequence, the infant may develop an abnormal dependency need, which can lead to an insatiable appetite or, conversely, to a refusal to eat. Thus, an unholy alliance of interactor and eater roles can adversely affect the rest of the personality, represented in this case by its aggregate of somatic roles. If these needs for appropriate nurturing remain unfulfilled, then the infant faces physiological and psychological distress.

The discussion of human beings as role recipients implies that primary roles, at least in their early developmental stages, are unconscious. That is to say, infants neither choose their roles nor decide when and where to take on certain roles. The primary roles appear in the early development of a fetus and function in an essentially instinctual manner during the early months of an infant's life. There is no research within the fields of role theory or drama therapy to support any specific stages of psychological development, so my comments at this juncture are somewhat speculative. Some of the research in social-cognitive development, however, especially that conducted by Selman, Lavin, and Brion-Meisels (1982), is broad and is discussed in part below.

THE HUMAN BEING AS ROLE TAKER

As I have already mentioned, the primary somatic roles are further developed as they are exposed to the social world. There exists a transitional phase between those roles that are given and those that are taken, so that the infant can learn to adapt to changing somatic, environmental, and social circumstances. For example, the eater role initially develops in the womb, where the fetus receives all nutrients automatically from the mother. When infants are born, they must actually engage with their mothers in order to eat. In doing so, they expand the eater role, which now depends upon a social interaction. At this early developmental stage, however, infants are merged with their mothers and view the breast or bottle as an extension of their own bodies. As such, this is a transitional period, because an infant has not fully separated from the mother and become aware of the distinction between the entity that is "me," and that which is the mother, the other, the "not me."

Once the separation between "me" and "not me" is made, role taking as such begins. Its earliest form is imitation, simple mimicry by the infant. Infants imitate role models whom they deem powerful. Their imitations of simple gestures, facial expressions, sounds, words, and actions mark a complex stage of development toward independence and separation from others. In imitating, one acts like the other, but to do so, paradoxically, one must first be able to see oneself as separate from the other. Thus, role taking begins in behavior reproduced from a powerful or competent role model. From an infant's point of view, one who can clap or smile or kiss is deemed powerful and competent.

The development of role taking proceeds from behavior to imagery as children internalize roles of significant others within their social environments. This occurs through a process of identification, the taking in of a desirable set of characteristics displayed by a role model. Taking in implies a continuity between the external world and one's inner experience. As the external world, represented by roles, is internalized, one's inner world, represented by a system of roles, expands. Through identification, one is able not only to take on another's perspective, but also to transform that perspective into one's own. For example, a nurturing mother serves as a role model for her young son and daughter. As both take on the role of nurturing mother, they will play it out later in relation to others, in their own unique fashion, based upon a variety of prevailing circumstances. Furthermore, by virtue of taking on that role, they will have the capacity to nurture themselves as their mother has nurtured them.

The developing child also takes on the role that G. H. Mead (1934) calls the "generalized other," that of the social group or organization. For example, young athletes first playing a team sport take on the generalized role of team, thus learning what they must do in their position in relation to others in theirs. Children take on the generalized role of parents, allowing them to understand what it means to be children in relationship to their families. As an example, my daughter, Georgie, began at 15 months of age to use the word "Daddy" with great regularity, as a means of identifying my role as her father and her complementary role of daughter. She omitted the word "Mommy" for reasons unknown, although it did affect her mother, who was anxious to be en-roled by her daughter. Perhaps she picked up on her mother's anxiety and fostered it as a way of distancing herself—that is, asserting her burgeoning independence.

By 16 months Georgie intoned "Daddy" and "Mommy," much to the delight of her mother, as she began to identify her parents as a generalized other. When she turned 17 months, she performed a curious ritual one evening. Her mother and I were sitting on opposite sides of the living room. In between us was a coffee table, and Georgie had taken up two miniature figures of familiar *Sesame Street* characters to play with at the table. After talking to them in a serious toddler babble, she proceeded to walk back and forth to her mother and me, touching each of us on the arm, body, and face while chanting "Mommy" or "Daddy" over and over again. After walking back and forth several times, she returned to the table and her small companions, and proceeded to speak to them, babbling again in a serious tone.

While watching this display, both of us commented that our daughter appeared to be telling her companions a story of who she was in relation to us as her parents. By touching both of us, Georgie made us real for herself. I was wearing glasses, and she would pat me there several times as she chanted, "Daddy, Daddy, Daddy," soon to shift to her mother's body and name. This naming of the significant others in her life was Georgie's way of taking on the generalized role of parents, and thus affirming her identity as daughter.

The extraordinary element in her dramatic play concerned the taking on of the storyteller role. Not only was she discovering a separation and connection between the social roles of daughter and parents, but also that between the intrapsychic roles of the active protagonist (the one who does the naming and has experiences) and the more passive narrator (the one who tells about the experiences she has had). In a sense, Georgie, in speaking to her imaginary audience, was learning the reflective role of the observer, who needs to make sense of her actions in some meaningful way. She was demonstrating to us in her dramatic play the beginnings of an imaginative life, marked by the ability to reflect upon her experience through story.

Individuals act in the world on the basis of the roles they have received and internalized. The alcoholic, the athlete, the son and daughter, the theatrical performer all act consistent in some ways with their internalized role models. When one procures a role from the social world, one tends to take on qualities of the model, rather than its totality. What qualities of the role model are taken on?

To begin with, certain physical qualities are taken: the demeanor of the parents, the gestures and sounds of the sibling, the swagger of the hero. In addition, cognitive styles, values and sensibilities, cultural, political, spiritual and socioeconomic points of view are taken on to some degree from the role model. The substance that is internalized, then, is quite complex, and serves to form one's own developing world view. The mix of images taken on as one internalizes the role of mother, for example, does not necessarily reproduce a copy of the role model. Sometimes a reflection results; at other times there is a refraction, a splitting of the mother role into several subroles. For example, a developing child may over time play out several versions of mother as nurturing and withholding, as loving and abusive, all based in diverse internalized qualities of actual or symbolic mothers.

The roles that are taken on from the social world are called "secondary roles," determined not by genetics but by social relationships. Secondary roles begin in imitation and proceed toward identification when children are more fully able to distinguish between themselves and others, the "me" and the "not me." This process is not strictly linear, as further imitation occurs long after the individual is capable of identification. Roles to be taken on belong initially to the domain of the "not me," like parts in a play. In the taking on of the social roles, actors in everyday life add further dimension to their role systems, the inner collection of roles that make up, in large part, their personalities. In juxtaposing the "not me" and the "me," individuals develop the ability to take on a wide variety of perspectives. The ultimate aim of role taking is to develop this ability fully by virtue of internalizing diverse perspectives.

Significant research related to this point has been conducted by Robert Selman and his colleagues at the Laboratory of Human Development at Harvard. Selman's work is modeled after the cognitive-developmental paradigm of Piaget (1926) and is very much based upon Mead's notion of role taking. His research has involved, among other things, developing an initial model of role taking, which has expanded into that of social perspective taking. Selman et al. (1982) specify five developmental stages through which one passes in taking on multiple points of view. The first, Stage 0, is that of egocentric or undifferentiated perspectives. At this stage, children from about 3 to 5 years old are unable to distinguish inner psychological states from outer experience in the world. At Stage 0 a sense of identity is based most fully on physical attributes.

Stage 1 is that of subjective or differentiated perspectives. Children from about 5 to 7 years old begin to recognize differences between inner and outer states, and thus distinctions between their own perspective and those of others. At Stage 2, that of self-reflective or reciprocal perspectives, children from approximately 7 to 11 years old are capable of assuming the point of view of another person and understanding the connection between another's thoughts and feelings and their own.

Stage 3, occurring during the pre-adolescent years, is that of third-person or mutual perspectives. At this point, children appear as both observers or subjects, and observed or objects; they are able to distance themselves from an interaction and to understand the different points of view of each interactor. At Stage 2 a child is more a passive observer, whereas at Stage 3 the child becomes "an active psychological manipulator of inner life" (Selman et al., 1982, p. 72).

Stage 4, the final stage of societal or in-depth perspectives, occurs during adolescence. Individuals are now able to understand that the taking on of mutual perspectives is based not only upon common interests, but sometimes upon unconscious processes that are not available to awareness. That is, differing points of view can be accepted on the basis of the knowledge that motives or needs are not necessarily subject to conscious awareness and rational explanation. Furthermore, mutual perspectives can become generalized to represent a societal or moral point of view.

Selman et al's system, within the tradition of cognitive and developmental psychology, is based upon the notion of a constructed self that in normal development becomes increasingly decentered—that is, less egocentric and more capable of taking on multiple perspectives. Although this constructivist point of view is useful in conceptualizing the process of role taking, it does so from a cognitive perspective and does not point to the connections among biology (roles given), cognition (roles taken), and action (roles played). Nor does it address the dramatic notion of role as a projection as well as construction, a mediator between the mind and the world.

Roles taken offer a kind of legacy that in many ways is related to roles given. It is unclear how much choice individuals, especially infants and children, have in taking on roles. It would appear that the taking on of sexual roles, for example, through an identification with the same- or opposite-sex parent, is automatic and unconscious. It would also appear that the taking on of certain psychological roles, such as that of the addict, occurs without much conscious choice, as if these were primary, somatic roles. This kind of role legacy is supported by research noting that alcoholism is passed from fathers to sons, whereas daughters of alcoholics tend to develop eating disorders, a form of substance abuse that is more common among females than males (U.S. Department of Health and Human Services, 1990; McFarland & Baker-Baumann, 1989). Perhaps this legacy is based upon a dual identification, in that these daughters take on the role of substance abuser from their fathers, but the substance of choice is more fully associated with their mothers. The role of the alcoholic, among others, then, although seemingly chosen, appears to be inherited within certain families.

Some roles taken are consciously chosen. Role taking and role choosing are not mutually exclusive processes. Both imply an identification with a role model and internalization of certain qualities of that model. Role choosing, however, suggests a conscious decision on the part of the person to take the desired qualities; for example, one may choose to model oneself after an athlete, a strong moral figure, or a successful criminal. Even in these examples, however, there is still the hint of an incipient legacy passed along over generations—if not through blood, then through socialization.

Role, then, is very much at the center of the personality. It is essentially a fluid sequence of traits, as well as a frame for and prelude to action. Role, as primary experience, is in some ways genetically programmed and somatically based. As secondary experience, that which is taken on, role intersects with one's social world through an external process of imitation and an internal process of identification with significant individual and generalized role models. Within the psychologically healthy person, there is a continuity between roles given and roles taken. Such a person tends to take on roles from the social world that complement or supplement given somatic roles.

Role assumes a third function, becoming action, when it is played out behaviorally.

THE HUMAN BEING AS ROLE PLAYER

Role by its nature can only assume fully visible form when enacted. Although the role played is only one realized aspect of the personality, it is the most accessible and overt one that is communicated to others and consequently judged by them.

The ability to play roles comes from one's need to assert oneself in the world. There are, in effect, as many explanations for why one plays roles as there are for why one plays. Let it suffice to speculate that one plays a role for two reasons. The first concerns a completion of the cycle of assimilation and accommodation so essential for cognitive development (see Piaget, 1952)—that is, adapting to the demands of one's environment on the basis of what one has internalized, and concurrently taking in the world on the basis of one's adaptations. In simple language, that which is inside must come out, and that which is outside must find a way back in, in order to become meaningful action. One plays a role, then, to get out of oneself, to locate a form for one's thought and feeling. In the role playing, the implicit thought and feeling are made explicit as they are transformed from mental images to actions. Conversely, through the role playing, one also internalizes further images that will guide later processes of assimilation and accommodation.

The second reason why one plays a role is to master it within an appropriate context. Playing out the role of father competently, for instance, implies the existence of children to be fathered. In many instances, a role calls out the role player and demands attention. For example, while I was in Greece, the role of searcher became activated and called itself forth from among the many other fearful roles that tend to dictate so much of my behavior. It was the searcher role that brought me to Mount Athos. This choosing of the person by the persona is not arbitrary, but arises from a particular context, whether that of family relationships or spiritual journeys. The external set of circumstances coincides with an inner readiness not only to act, but to act competently—to master a bit of reality that has heretofore been beyond one's grasp.

One plays roles, then, primarily to get in and out of oneself and to master both that which is situated inside, the role taken, and outside, the objective world. The more competently one plays out one's roles, the more one will develop an ease in navigating the sometimes difficult boundaries between internal and external experience.

When role playing becomes dysfunctional,* an individual loses the ability to move freely between internal subjective experience and the external world. For some, the boundaries between the two states become too diffuse, leading to a confusion of a dream state with a waking state, fantasy with reality. Or the boundaries may become too rigid, implying a denial of either the imaginative life or the social one. Dysfunctional role playing is often marked by a lack of role ambivalence, leading one to retreat into a minimum of nonthreatening roles, or by an overabundance of role ambivalence, leading to a confusion among roles. In either case, the roles played are not mastered but rather appear to master the role player, to the extent that they overpower the entire role system.

An acquaintance whom I shall call Sam, exemplified the unambivalent man who appeared to live in a factual and literal world for 90 years, devoid of dreams and possibilities. Knowing the man to be one who might say, with T. S. Eliot's (1915/1963) J. Alfred Prufrock, "I have measured out my life with coffee spoons," I took interest in the fact that Sam had kept a daily journal for 70 years. When I asked to see what he had written, he opened up his carefully labeled volumes. In a meticulous hand he had transcribed the minutiae of each day: the meals eaten, the family members who came and went, the phone calls received, the weather, and above all, the various costs of things. There was little or no mention of the dramatic events of world wars, assassinations, shifts in lifestyles and political systems, and the consequences of births and deaths in the family. Sam transcribed the facts. His was a diary without a commentary. For this J. Alfred Prufrock, unmarried and childless, things were as they appeared to be.

Sam's apparently one-dimensional life seemed consistent with his occupational role of accountant, which he played out over 65 years. When he died, his accounts were all settled, his journal complete. Yet his last years were bitter and angry, spent railing against the cruelty of his relatives who (he claimed) had abandoned him to his growing infirmities, even as they waited for him to die and leave his

---

*Functional versus dysfunctional role playing is difficult to assess precisely, although some attempts have been made (see Johnson, 1988). This issue is further addressed in a discussion of diagnostic implications of the role method.

presumed fortune in their greedy hands. As such, Sam felt very much the victim.

Sam had grown up in poverty and worked obsessively to support many in his family. He worked his way through college and struggled through the Great Depression to survive. His role models were those industrious souls who knew how to save (and squeeze) a penny. Like many from Eastern European immigrant families, he bought fully into the American dream that rewards enterprise and individualism, but ignores a sense of social responsibility.

This rigid man, miserly to the extreme, intolerant and insulated from the dangers of the outside world, was, however, a survivor. He did reminisce and tell stories with a noticeable twinkle in his eye to those few willing to listen. I was one of them, and when I visited Sam I would encourage the storyteller part of him. His stories presented a cast of victims and aggressors, heroes and villains, all based upon family members. The most bitter portrayals were of those who either neglected or patronized him, waiting for a big payoff upon his death. I wondered whether it was these stories, in part, that had kept him going throughout 90 years, providing something beyond the drabness of the literal.

Sam died angry and isolated. He left behind a will that meticulously discriminated among the remaining family members, much to their dismay. This final document told a bizarre story about old family squabbles, forgotten visits, and telephone calls never made. In its own way, it displayed the roles he could never play out in his lifetime: family patriarch and provider, judge and jury, avenger. Above all, Sam's will was a joke on those who assumed they would inherit his money by virtue of playing out their family roles to his satisfaction; in death, he played the trickster. He finally told his story, reaching with a great leap of the imagination far beyond the literalness of his life.

Sam's case illustrates that even in the life of a man whose existence by most standards was sorely lacking in diversity and joy, there are other aspects of the personality that may be submerged as unenacted roles. In this case, such roles were strong enough to be unleashed after death.

On the other side of the spectrum is a client of mine, Kate, the complete actor. For Kate, nothing is literal. She tells me her dreams as if she were describing an outing taken the day before. Her multidimensionality is overwhelming as she speaks of her many lovers, her journeys to exotic countries, her several marriages and seven children, her theatrical roles and psychotherapeutic training, her visits with shamans and witches—all within her 50 years. Kate has fashioned a lifestyle for herself that allows her to survive by taking on odd jobs in theatre, journalism, education, and psychotherapy. But she has also split herself into so many pieces that she has ended up more than once in the psychiatric hospital.

Speaking with Kate is an adventure. She is highly articulate and imaginative, and is often several steps beyond the logic of those with whom she attempts to communicate. However, despite her fine performance in many of her professional and personal roles, Kate's ability to maintain a sense of equilibrium often escapes her. She seems at best to just get by. Unable to maintain a job, she tends to flit from one vocational role to another. She is in chronic financial debt and at times feels overwhelmed by her lack of stability.

Kate is a wanderer without a clear sense of destination. The roles she plays, although consistent with those she has taken in, are likely to be inconsistent with the roles demanded by the outside world. Most often, she disregards the social context completely. Although her life is rich in fantasy and profoundly different from Sam's, her dilemma is all too similar: an encroaching resentment toward a world that has not rewarded her special talents; a fear of slipping toward old age with little power and control.

Sam, a man with too few roles, and Kate, a woman with too many, took many years to develop their role systems and to fashion their behaviors in role. As dysfunctional role players, they were generally unable or unwilling to critically assess how well or poorly they were (and, in Kate's case, are) served by their roles. Thus, their developing behaviors in role tended to take control of their lives.

Was Sam's role as tight-fisted, miserly accountant really his only means of self-expression? And has Kate's expansive role repertoire really mitigated against the possibility of her playing out a single role with competence and mastery? I think not. Sometimes it takes an outside event—a sudden change in status, for example—for one to expand a limited repertoire or to assume a single role more competently. For Sam, the shift came as he prepared for his death. For Kate, that shift was manifest when she was surprisingly thrust into the new role of grandmother. She not only devoted herself to her granddaughter, but also found a new meaning in her mother role.

As mentioned above, role development implies some degree of ambivalence within roles, between roles, and as an existential condition. The fully one-dimensional being does not exist in human form, so long as consciousness and the ability to distinguish between "me" and "not me" is available. Role development also implies the possibility of change or shift in one's constellation of roles. Even as ambivalences are played out and shifts occur, there appears to be a stable system that holds together the often contradictory and changing roles.

If roles are personae, this system may be seen as the personality. More in keeping within a dramatic framework, this structure can be conceptualized as the "role system."

THE ROLE SYSTEM

Individual roles, such as the miserly isolate and the free-spirited wanderer, can be organized according to given categories and criteria within those categories. In subsequent chapters I construct such a system in the form of a taxonomy, drawing my categories of role from both theatre and everyday life. At any given time, depending upon a particular context, one role or a configuration of several related roles may become prominent. I have noted above that Sam, preparing for his death, mobilized both playful and vindictive roles as his last act of will. And I have described in the Introduction how the related roles of hero and coward became activated as I moved toward and within the community of Mount Athos. When this occurs, those internal roles that have little connection to, for example, the terrors and joys of the journey remain temporarily dormant. However, they are ready to be activated at a moment's notice. When a trickster appears in the spiritual environment, one may need a warrior role in defense. When a holy man appears, one may need a cautious part, again for protection, or perhaps a believer part to unfold oneself to the spiritual dimension of the meeting.

A role system is built on the interplay between complementary roles, such as wife and mother, and between a role and its counterpart(s), such as victim and survivor. Within the system, one category of roles (e.g., spiritual roles) intersects with others (e.g., social roles). In the taxonomy developed in this book, six broad categories of role are delineated: somatic, cognitive, affective, social, spiritual, and aesthetic.

The role system serves as a frame for primary roles, those given; secondary roles, those taken; and tertiary roles, those played out. One's role system contains individual roles, such as the fool, and their qualitatively unique subroles, such as the trickster and the clown.

As one grows older, one's role system generally expands in complexity. The primary, somatic roles, though fixed in quantity, tend to change in quality as they interact with secondary and tertiary roles. The role of the eater, for example, changes from infancy to childhood as the child begins to internalize a role model who may be on a special diet.

Generally speaking, the complexity of one's role system depends upon the quantity of roles taken. With this internal complexity, one has greater potential to play out a greater variety of roles. This notion is based upon favorable environmental circumstances—that is, a heterogeneous society comprised of differing points of view. Role quality is equally important in personality development as one identifies with given social, moral, and political role models. In moving from an egocentric to a decentered stance, the developing individual should be able to assume varying social, moral, and political perspectives that provide a qualitative sense of identity.

A role system, then, is made up of interdependent roles, which can be organized in categories that are themselves interrelated. Even when the person is at rest, one or a related series of roles will tend to predominate in the personality, causing other categories or individual roles to recede. With disuse or neglect, these roles tend to become dormant, to the extent that the person may forget that they even existed at all. Such hidden roles may become activated by a sudden crisis (e.g., when one is faced with a life-threatening disease) or more gradually (e.g., as one passes through a further developmental stage, through a self-reflective or psychotherapeutic process, or through a significant relationship with another human being).

Any single change of role that is qualitatively significant will affect the whole role system—for example, becoming a parent for the first time, or working through the dysfunctional role of victim in therapy and becoming more assertive in dealing with others. A healthy role system is a flexible one that has room for these kinds of changes and can support role ambivalences that seem to lie at the foundation of each role system. Each role is subject to any number of pulls and pushes, accidental and planned blessings and curses. And each role system, if healthy, has the flexibility to expand and contract when necessary to accommodate the infinite physiological and psychological shifts that occur in a person's life.

A role system contains the substance of one's identity—all the pieces that, once assembled, represent a personality. However, this system is perpetually in flux, changing according to one's experiences within the somatic and social environments. As such, this assembly is impossible to view objectively.

An underlying assumption of this book is that roles can be modified at any stage of development—whether as a child, adolescent, adult, or elder—by working through the paradigm of the primary roles that are genetically given, the secondary roles that are socially taken, and the tertiary roles that are behaviorally played out. In later chapters, I specify those roles that are available to be given, taken on, and played out. But, first, let us see how the concept of role can be translated into a clinical method of treatment through drama therapy.

CHAPTER THREE

The Drama Therapy
Role Method

Drama therapy is distinct among other forms of psychotherapy in that it proceeds through role. That is, both client and therapist take on and play out roles in order to help the client discover and/or recover the most functional role system.

A number of approaches have been devised that guide the treatment process in drama therapy. One, the developmental approach (see Johnson, 1982, 1991), is based primarily on an object relations model and views the work as proceeding from lower- to higher-order competencies as expressed through sound, movement, and verbalization. Another approach is that of storytelling and storymaking (see Gersie, & King, 1990; Gersie 1991), which is based on a narrative model and helps clients make sense of their lives through identifying with the themes and structures of classical and personal stories. A third approach, stemming from a social-anthropological model (see Jennings, 1993), examines the ritual and cultural aspects of everyday life and helps clients re-examine their belief systems through metaphorical and symbolic means.

Most other approaches tend to be derivative of psychoanalytical play therapy (see Irwin, 1983) or various forms of improvised drama (see Emunah, 1993) and performed theatre (see Jennings, 1990). Those who practice dramatic play therapy adapt the classical approaches of Melanie Klein (1932), Margaret Lowenfeld (1979), and Virginia Axline (1947), among others, to the needs of particular clients. Those who practice improvisational or theatrical forms base their work on an aesthetic model, adapting their dramatic methods to meet psychotherapeutic goals.

The role method in drama therapy admits the value of all these approaches, but attempts to further systematize what it views as the primary component of healing through the art form of drama—that of role. The healing potential of role is to be found as it positions the role taker or role player within the dramatic paradox of "me" and "not me." The therapeutic actor, like the theatrical actor, is given permission to move in and out of two contiguous realities: that of the imagination, the source of unconscious imagery, and that of the everyday, the domain of grounded daily existence. While in the transitional space (see Winnicott, 1971) between the two realities, the actor is capable of both viewing a problematic issue and working it through.

The role method as described here evolved inductively, through many years of clinical work with clients and experimentation with training groups of graduate students and professionals. It further developed as I contemplated the dramatic connection, conceiving of theatre as a repository of repeated role types, functions, and styles. The role method, as a means of treatment, involves eight steps:

1. Invoking the role.
2. Naming the role.
3. Playing out/working through the role.
4. Exploring alternative qualities in subroles.
5. Reflecting upon the role play: discovering role qualities, functions, and styles inherent in the role.
6. Relating the fictional role to everyday life.
7. Integrating roles to create a functional role system.
8. Social modeling: discovering ways that clients' behavior in role affects others in their social environments.

THE INVOCATION OF THE ROLE

One's role system is fully portable. At any given time it can be accessed, yet few people would think to check in with their internal cast of characters. Furthermore, one's role system changes continually, depending upon time, place, and need. Thus, a woman serving in the army may play the role of nurturing mother while at home but then play the fearless soldier when required to fight in a war far away from home. This particular example was highlighted by the news media during the Persian Gulf war, when American women entered combat situations, some losing their lives.

In drama therapy, a role is invoked by helping a client reach into the system and extract one that needs to be expressed and examined. The role is invoked as a way to help the client immediately focus upon a single aspect of personality. The invocation, like that of a poet invoking the muse, is a means of inspiration. Through calling forth one part of the personality, the client seeks inspiration. That part will guide the client, hopefully, to the source of an issue that needs to be addressed.

The invocation of the role, then, is a calling into being of that part of the person that will inspire a creative search for meaning. Within the role method, the invocation usually proceeds unconsciously; that is, clients will not be asked directly to choose a role that they think is important, but rather to engage in a creative process that will lead to the invocation of a role. For example, I often begin drama therapy groups with a movement warm-up, asking all to move freely throughout the space. Then, I ask the clients to focus upon one part of their bodies and to allow a movement to extend from that source; for example, a prominent belly may lead to a slow and heavy movement. From there, I ask people to extend their movements further and allow a character to emerge from the belly.

Once the character is clearly visible, the invocation is complete. If the client has worked spontaneously without predetermining who and what the character should be, then the role has indeed emerged from an unconscious source. In some ways the role actually chooses the role player: It highlights an issue, often not consciously accessible to the client, that needs to be addressed at that moment. In some instances, clients may be fully conscious of problematic roles. They may have entered drama therapy in the first place because of the nagging persistence of their victim role, for example. In such cases, when the role is already present, clients begin at the next step—naming the role.

THE NAMING OF THE ROLE

Once the role is invoked, it needs to be further substantiated through naming. The client may give the role a reality-based name, such as Sam or Sarah, or a more abstract or poetic one. The belly character may become Hound Dog, for example. Or the naming may well correspond to a prescribed role type (e.g., The Bully or The Coward). Michael, the subject of the case discussed in Chapters Four and Five, named the angry part of himself Black Rage.

Naming is important, in that it helps the client further concretize the chosen role. The naming also allows clients to move away from their daily reality into the fictional, creative realm. Some clients, especially those who are too close to their problems and/or too restrictive in their ability to play, will impose their actual names upon the role. In that case, they should be encouraged to fictionalize the role through choosing another name. In doing so, they take a significant step into the paradox of the dramatic process: of being oneself and not oneself at the same time.

Naming is a means of making a choice that has certain implications. For example, some people will call their angry parts gentle or weak names. One client referred to the furious part of herself as Passive; by implication, this was a person unable to admit her angry feelings. In extreme cases when anger is turned inward, the clients will commit self-destructive acts. In choosing anonymity or suicide, they take a radical approach to resolving the ambivalence of being. One client, unable to express anger and fearful of becoming invisible, named her angry role Suomy Nona— "Anonymous" spelled backward.

In choosing a name for a role, a client dares to look at the connection between a feeling state and a behavioral state. For example, a client who feels angry but behaves passively may well experience anxiety when faced with provocative situations. The naming, then, forces the issue of examining contradictions between appearance and reality. Furthermore, the naming allows one to play with fantasies of superior strength, beauty, courage, and intellect; this leads to a search for the connection between the ideal and the real.

In the balcony scene in Shakespeare's *Romeo and Juliet* (1595/1959), Juliet asks, "What's in a name?" When she continues, "That which we call a rose/By any other name would smell as sweet" (Act II, scene ii, 43–44), she is only partly accurate. Names are loaded with implication, as any expectant parent about to decide upon a name for the new baby knows. If the rose were called "skunk," one would not expect it to smell as sweet, and thus it probably wouldn't. Or one might not even attempt to smell the rose at all.

A role like that of the hothead by any other name, such as Passive, is equally suspect. In the role method, the client is challenged to commit to a name that seems right at that time. The working through of the implications of that commitment follows.

THE PLAYING OUT/WORKING THROUGH OF THE ROLE

In a group drama therapy situation, each member at this stage has at least one role available. The next logical step is to deepen a sense of that role through various forms of enactment. In some cases individuals will be asked to work in front of the group, creating stories or monologues from the point of view of their characters. In many cases individuals will work together, collectively improvising a scene or dramatizing a story, all in role.

The working-through stage is a time of enhancing one's commitment to a role and extending it beyond expected behaviors. One client, Ellen, in the role of Emily, the perfectionist, engaged in a series of enactments in group, one of which was a dinner table scene in which all clients took on the roles of members of a fictional family. In playing the perfectionist, she began to discover ways that Emily overpowered the family through judgment and sarcasm, and to realize how those qualities kept her ultimately from satisfying her deeper needs for acceptance and love.

In individual therapy, a similar process occurs after a client has identified and named a significant and problematic role. Much of the actual therapy concerns a working through of the issues embedded in a particular role (or related roles). In Chapters Four and Five, the case of Michael illustrates how an individual worked through a number of roles, including adolescent, gay man, son, hothead, hypochondriac, and victim. In this case, Michael's primary means of work was through storytelling.

Michael's example is significant in that during actual drama therapy, a client does not simply focus upon a single role and work it through until the process is concluded. In fact, clients often move from role to role, shifting focus as needed. From the therapist's point of view, it is important to try to help the clients look at the implications of such shifts. Are they shifting because they are unable or unwilling to work with a single role, one that might be too threatening? Or are they shifting because they are examining a system of interdependent roles and need the freedom to maneuver among them?

The working through is generally the action segment of the therapy, preceded by the first two steps, which provide a warm-up to the action. Working through occurs in role and is most successful when clients are able to fully accept the fictional reality of the drama. The consequences of enactment during this stage accrue to the characters as opposed to the actors. During the working-through stage, then, the actors are potentially free to experiment with their roles. For example, a woman can experiment with the role of pariah, knowledgeable that it is not she who has risked her life by living on the fringes of society, but some alter ego, another rose (being) of a different name.

EXPLORING ALTERNATIVE QUALITIES IN SUBROLES

When I began training drama therapists in 1980, I devised an approach that I called the "extended dramatization" —a 30-hour experience (15 sessions lasting 2 hours each) in working through a drama therapy process. During the first hour, every one in the group was to invoke and then name a single role. Throughout the first 20 hours, they played out and worked through those roles. However, after the completion of 10 hours, they were asked to create one modification of the initial role, and then a second that also stemmed from the original character.

The first additional role was to be in the form of a puppet, representing a subtype—a variation on the theme set by the character, in order to provide it with further dimension and specificity. The second was to be in the form of a mask, representing a second thematic variation, more extreme in its divergence from the initial role. The alternative quality of the mask was to be one that had not been expressed openly at all within the dramatization.

Initially, many trainees would express distress at having to stay with one role for 30 hours, especially those who chose a threatening or limited one. And invariably, they would feel a sense of relief at being able to extend the one into the many. Exploring alternatives is important because the actors begin to recognize options and work with them. In many ways, this allows them to work through their ambivalences toward their roles.

As an example, Joan called her initial role Iphigenia. She quickly became aware of the fact that she was working with the role of victim, who, like the classical Iphigenia, had lost all control of her life and had no choice but to give up her life for the good of the community. Having worked through her victim role for some 10 hours, she created a puppet that she named The Martyr. As a subtype of victim (26.1 in the taxonomy; see Chapter Nine and the Appendix), the martyr embodies the quality of self-sacrifice, rather than simply giving oneself up to the control of someone else. Through working with The Martyr as puppet, Joan began to see the dilemma of the martyr subtype, who is victimized by, in fact, choosing to sacrifice her well-being for the sake of others.

Finally, in building her mask, Joan was able to extend her understanding further. The mask character, which she named The Mother, became one who sacrificed her self-interests in order to manipulate others by saying things like this: "How can you treat me this way after all I've done for you? I gave up everything I had so that you could live a better life than mine!" The Mother was a selfish, guilt-inspiring manipulator, more victimizer than victim (the self-serving martyr; 26.2 in the taxonomy).

Joan was able to move toward these discoveries as she worked through two sub-types of the victim, that of martyr and its alternative, the self-serving martyr, one who inspires guilt by pretending to have truly sacrificed her well-being.

Most work with subroles does not fit so precisely within the drama therapy role model. However, as a way of working, the use of subroles allows clients to dig deeper within their characters. On that dig, most will discover that any role, when explored fully, embodies contradictions and ambivalences. The role method encourages the search for those ambivalences, even as an initial role (like that of the victim) shifts to its apparent opposite (that of the victimizer). Once the alternatives have been unearthed, they too should be named, so that the clients can move on to the next stage in the process—making sense of the role play.

REFLECTING UPON THE ROLE PLAY

The next several steps involve what is traditionally known as the "closure," the time for stepping back from the actual drama and discussing its meaning. Closure is a way not only of helping clients assess the value of the drama, but also of validating their feelings and providing needed transitions from the world of the imagination to that of the here and now, and from the contained therapy space to the less controlled space of everyday life.

Within the role method, the first part of the closure involves the ability to find meaning in the roles and subroles played from the fictional point of view. Joan, described just above, was asked generally: "How does Iphigenia play out her victim role within your drama?" Her focus was upon the role, and thus she was able to maintain a degree of safe distance, as she was not required to speak directly about herself.

More specifically, clients can be asked to specify the physical, intellectual, moral, emotional, social, spiritual, and/or aesthetic qualities of their roles. This can be done in an informal, anecdotal fashion, related to the function of the character. Examples of the kinds of questions that can be addressed are as follows: How do the physical qualities of the character (e.g., the prominent belly) help to shape his behavior and sense of well-being? How does Iphigenia feel as victim? Does she see herself as a self-sacrificing martyr or as a guilt-inspiring one? What is the purpose of her suffering? If there is a spiritual quality about her, how does it help her cope with her victim role?

During this stage, the clients are also asked to speak about their style of enactment. For example, was Iphigenia played broadly and abstractly, moving away from the more emotional element of her role?

Or was she portrayed realistically, providing a heartfelt view of her dilemma as victim? What are the implications of playing a role one way or the other? Does the use of presentational style allow the client the safety to reveal personal issues? Or does it provide a means to resist the search for feeling?

Thus, the discussion focuses upon the importance of how a role is played, of the connection between feeling and thought. When the purpose and form of the role are clear, then it is time to proceed to the next step.

RELATING THE FICTIONAL ROLE
TO EVERYDAY LIFE

Ultimately, all forms of projective therapy are successful to the extent that they lead the client into and out of the projection. In the case of drama therapy, the projective work involves, first, a movement from an everyday, ordinary role into an imaginative, dramatic one. Thus, Joan, the client, took on the role of Iphigenia, the victim.

During the preceding step, Joan was asked to examine the quality, function, and style of Iphigenia within the fictional drama she created. Now Joan was asked to return from the reality of the imagination to that of the everyday, and to look at the connections between the two. Joan's primary questions during this stage became: "How am I like Iphigenia?", and the converse, "How am I different from Iphigenia?" The latter became important in demonstrating that Joan's whole personality, represented by her role system, was larger than any one role she might play.

Assuming that the clients are already aware of the qualities, functions, and style of their fictional role, this next step returns them to their own reality and challenges them to look at ways that they play the role in their interactions with others. For some, the connection is difficult to see. Another woman playing a martyr role might have created a broad, caricatured martyr that bore little resemblance to her own life. In discussion, this client would be asked to specify the qualities, function, and style of her own daily martyr role to determine how it serves her. Then she would be asked to compare that to the fiction she created. Should the fictional martyr prove more powerful and liberating, then client and therapist would discuss ways of bringing some of its qualities and stylistic elements into the everyday experience of playing the martyr.

In many ways, the therapist functions as a theatre director, attempting to help an actor find a way to connect personal experience with the demands of a scripted character. The main difference is that in theatre, the personal serves the fictional; in therapy, the fictional serves the personal. In a more integral, poetic sense, however, both serve each other, as art sometimes mirrors nature and nature sometimes mirrors art.

To discover meaning in a fictional role, a client must be able to accept the dramatic paradox of person and persona and find a way to live in an ambivalent world of being and not being. Thus, the fictional role serves the client by pointing to an equivalent nonfictional role. That role, in turn, requires the fiction for elucidation. The dramatic mirror has two sides, both of which refer to the other, and either of which is meaningless without the other.

To understand how my fictional roles serve me in my everyday life, then, I must be able to see both fictional role and its reality-based counterpart clearly, comprehending the content, purpose, and form of each. Furthermore, I need to examine the differences and similarities between them. And finally, I need to look toward modifying the everyday role in such a way that it serves me as well as or better than the fictional one. Only then can I begin to see the intimate connection between the real and ideal, the true and the false, the substance and the shadow—all providing sustenance to each other even as they feed upon each other.

INTEGRATING ROLES TO CREATE A FUNCTIONAL ROLE SYSTEM

The actual process of drama therapy does not necessarily proceed in such a neat, linear fashion, according to these given steps. In fact, some clients generate several roles during a given session. Others, having invoked, named, and begun to work through a single role, often become sidetracked by other roles that are either fully or dimly perceived. Some of these will also need to be named and worked through to a certain extent. One's focus upon a role fades in and out according to one's immediate and/or past experience, mood, resistance, and motivation.

That notwithstanding, the role method is still valuable as a map to help the client and drama therapist specify and then traverse often obscure territory. The ultimate goal in its use is to help the client construct a viable role system—one that is able to tolerate ambivalence and acknowledge the importance of both negative and positive roles.

In moving toward the conclusion of a successful therapeutic process, a client comes to recognize how the various roles taken and played work together. Joan, for example, began to realize how the victim worked with the victimizer, and in particular how the mother worked with the daughter, using the guilt-inducing martyr quality as a means of controlling the daughter's need for liberation and playfulness. She further began to remove the blame for her victim-like persona from an external source, her mother, as she realized that she had been mothering herself poorly. As she had taken on the martyr/mother configuration from her actual mother, so could she move toward a new sense of mothering herself—substituting self-satisfaction for self-sacrifice.

Roles tend to become entangled in one another. During the process of working through the role method, the client is challenged to unravel some of the knots and separate one role from the other. At the stage of integration, the system is reassembled but with specific roles transformed. The victim role, for Joan, was no longer what it had been in terms of quality and function. Its style had even shifted in the course of the treatment from the poetic, abstract silence and acceptance played out through the fictional Iphigenia, to the more heartfelt anger later expressed directly by Joan in her refusal to perpetuate acts of self-sacrifice.

Integration as an aim is often difficult to assess within the course of drama therapy. It occurs when there are some discernible shifts, as reported by the client. For Joan, it began in part with the rise of the hothead role and the demise of the martyr one. It continued as other roles became implicated—the mother, the moralist, and the immoralist, among others. In learning to mother herself, Joan was able to sustain an intimacy with a partner in such a way as to ask for and receive forms of caring and nurturance that she never before thought she deserved. She still had a tendency to be too quick to sacrifice her needs in order to avoid some imagined war, but learned more and more to catch herself before doing so.

Integration, though often difficult to specify, implies a reconfiguring of one's role system, so that, for example, the roles of victim and victor are in balance. The proof of the shift of roles can be seen in the ability to live with role ambivalence without undue distress and to discover new possibilities of being with oneself and others.

SOCIAL MODELING

Cycles of incest, neglect, violence, and addiction tend to run in families. Socially-based family roles often prove to be determinants of behavior that are as powerful as primary, somatic ones. Through the process of therapy, individuals seek ways of breaking the pattern. It seems to me that abusive patterns can be averted not only if the victims work through an abusive role and reconfigure their role system, but also if they are able to provide new models for intimates or dependents who would otherwise take on the abusive role.

Change of role system, then, is not enough. That is generally an internal matter. The clients must be able to play out a revised version of a dysfunctional role in order to influence others within their social sphere. Even when a role system shifts, the dysfunctional role still remains very much in existence, though in a less powerful state. In modeling the role of benign authority figure, for example, a person does not deny the part that is tyrannical and brutal, but tempers it with care and openness to dependents. Only then may a new order emerge. An alcoholic is always an alcoholic, but the power of that one role can be diminished as other, less dependent ones, such as the helper, the elder, and the orthodox believer, are developed and modeled. Within 12-step programs such as Alcoholics Anonymous, this notion is practiced daily. For many recovering alcoholics and others addicted to various substances, a great deal of hope springs from the reality of being part of a community of peers, some of whom have been able to transform their dependent, addictive roles. As such, these are the role models to be emulated by those so much in need of transformation.

The dramatic role method is a form of treatment. As mentioned above, it is not intended to be a rigid, linear system, but rather a set of guidelines. It offers a means of identifying role types and subtypes, qualities, functions, and styles. In practice, one does not need to focus upon all of these aspects in order to prove effective in helping people reconfigure their role systems and become positive role models themselves. Yet, as we shall see, the role method well informs the general process of treatment through drama therapy.

The case described in the next two chapters, that of Michael, proceeded through such a process. Again, it did not follow the exact chronology of the prescribed steps. But it did reflect a way of working that was consistent with the intent of both the role method as described here and the taxonomy of roles to be described in later chapters.

CHAPTER FOUR

The Case of Michael:
Part I

My work with Michael proceeded through a variety of drama therapy techniques, all involving a movement in and out of fictional roles. With the distance provided by the fiction, Michael was able to access rather deep levels of internal experience. Through this process, many roles within his role system were invoked, and problematic roles were worked through and integrated, leading to a revised role system. The primary approach in helping Michael reconfigure his role system was through stories, a number of which are told here. My interpretive comments are limited to a delineation of role types presented, and the qualities and functions of those roles. When appropriate, I also address Michael's style of role playing. Because drama therapy is generally a nonanalytical, creative form of treatment, I refrain from engaging in overly analytical commentary, allowing the process to unfold mainly in narrative form and couching my interpretations in the specified role model. Whenever possible, I let Michael speak for himself, as he was the author, actor, and ultimately healer of his several dramatic dilemmas.

BACKGROUND

When Michael began treatment, he was a 27-year-old gay man from an upper-middle-class suburb of Chicago. He was the middle child, with an older brother and a younger sister. He was thin, of medium height, and physically attractive; he dressed informally, often projecting a childlike or adolescent quality. When I first met him, he rarely established eye contact and often remained aloof. Michael was highly verbal, intelligent, and analytical concerning himself and others. He also had a tendency to be judgmental. Furthermore, he had a great need to express his feelings, although he would not do so unless he felt completely safe.

Upon graduating from college, Michael hoped to realize his dream of becoming a professional stage actor. Enrolling in a number of acting classes and performing in several small theatres, Michael worked hard to perfect his craft. Because his few acting jobs did not pay the bills, Michael supported himself as a temporary worker in various city office buildings. He devalued economic success, conceiving of himself as an artist—a role that did not require money and status, but simply important, challenging work. This role was in marked contrast to that of the affluent upper-middle-class boy raised in the suburbs, a role he still held onto. Michael returned home to his family in Chicago regularly, where he would eat and sleep a lot, and generally revisit his past as a means of delaying his fall into adulthood.

Michael began therapy because he felt fearful, isolated, and lonely a good deal of the time. He chose drama therapy because he often used words defensively to avoid feelings, and felt that he could express himself more authentically through a creative process. Michael often complained of psychosomatic illnesses. He manifested an intense fear of bugs, as well as a more reality-based fear of AIDS. Throughout the first 2 years of therapy, he did not have an AIDS test out of a paradoxical fear of dying and living.

As a gay male, Michael recognized a certain pain that comes from being a pariah. He saw his homosexuality as predetermined as opposed to willful. Men attracted him sexually; women did not. Yet he enjoyed friendship and intimacy with women. Of his siblings, he was much more attached his sister than to his brother. When he initially spoke of effeminate men, he became angry. The thought of being alone with a group of gay men threatened him. Michael was on a search to rediscover and integrate the feminine part of himself, left behind in his childhood play with dolls and female roles.

Michael had few sexual relationships, all of which tended to leave him with an empty, used feeling. He relied on anonymous telephone sex connections to satisfy some of his erotic needs. For these reasons, and because he had developed a strong AIDS consciousness, Michael was not very promiscuous. When sexually active, he practiced safe sex and strongly criticized anyone who did not.

When I first began to work with Michael, he identified very much with the role of innocent child who communed with nature and managed to stay clear of the evils of the adult world of experience and responsibility. The innocent role served to isolate Michael from both the adult parts of himself and from his peers who might carry the dis-ease of adult life.

Michael also conceived of himself as an abused child in relation to his father, who had beaten and humiliated him when he was a small boy. His relationship to his father became a central focus of his treatment. Michael's father was a successful businessman, although, according to Michael, he had inherited a thriving business from his in-laws. He was affable, highly social, and macho. He was also an exhibitionist who walked around naked not only in front of his family, but also in the presence of his children's friends. Such a display always humiliated Michael. Michael had early memories of being in bed with his mother while his father did pushups, naked, on the floor.

When Michael began therapy he appeared to be particularly merged with his sister, Bea, 25 years old, the youngest in the family. They shared the same sensibility and, most importantly, the same sense of humor. (Humor was what kept the family afloat, although it was often used as a defense against expressing direct feeling.) Michael expected Bea to love him unconditionally and wanted her all to himself. He was jealous of her successful heterosexual relationships with men, even though she seemed unable to sustain relationships. Michael saw Bea as beautiful though masculine in her demeanor.

Generally, Michael felt ambivalent toward his mother, whom he saw as unfeminine and withholding. On the one hand, she fed him, literally stuffing him with food and gifts when he returned home, and hugging him in a way that his father never could. On the other hand, she easily distanced herself from Michael and did not rescue him from the abuses of his father. Moreover, the mother's nurturing touch could easily become too intrusive and suffocating. Michael felt that he had inherited a negative legacy from her—a judgmental, perfectionistic quality that stood in the way of intimacy with others. He was able to confront his mother on occasion, when he was the object of her judgment. They fought often, accusing each other of small transgressions. Although there were many taboo subjects, the germ of a passionate connection existed between mother and son.

Michael's role of brother to his older male sibling, Steve, was much less developed than his relationship to Bea. Michael pictured him in the image of the father. He was fully masculine but also incomplete in the sense of understanding and dealing with the family dynamics. Michael felt that Steve would marry a woman like their mother.

From my point of view, Michael's role system was quite restricted. He did have a number of roles available, but they were often deflated and immature. The initial roles presented appeared to be primarily those of needy child, victim, and isolate.

BEGINNINGS

I first met Michael in a drama therapy workshop I conducted. We were working with stories, and he chose "Beauty and the Beast." After recounting the story, members of the group were asked to select one role with which they felt most identified. Michael chose the ring, which is a gift given to Beauty by her father. When the father offers Beauty to the Beast in exchange for his life, the daughter accepts her role gracefully. After staying with the Beast for some time, she requests that he allow her to visit her father and sisters once more before her father dies. The Beast agrees, but sets terms: a time limit and a tangible sign that she will return. That sign, her bond, is the ring.

At the conclusion of the workshop, Michael spoke of his connection to the ring role. It allowed him to become full of feeling, particularly love for his father. As the ring, he experienced a sense of peace.

Several months following the workshop, Michael and I began to work in individual drama therapy. During the first session, he again brought up the story of "Beauty and the Beast" and his attraction to the ring role.

I thought of a diminutive Samuel Beckett play, *Come and Go* (1968), an abstract piece involving three women who engage in esoteric rituals of entering, gossiping, and exiting. At the end, all hold hands as one of the women says, "I can feel the rings." I once directed the play and had some sense of the rings as bonds—racial, feminine ties. But none of these images fully satisfied me. The ring role remained mysterious, and so did Michael's invocation of the ring. In the story, it appears to be the bond to the father, who violates the bond by trading the daughter's life for his own. Yet it also represents a connection between Beauty and the Beast. Is it a transitional object that helps Beauty break with the father and move toward the lover? Or does it point toward the triangulation of father–daughter–lover (further complicated by the duality of Beast–lover), a psychological dilemma close to the spirit of Freud's Oedipus complex? I also wondered whether this Oedipal triangulation was a source of Michael's malaise.

Michael spoke rapidly and analytically during the first session.

He spoke of his need to feel, but tended to remain emotionally distant. He spoke of his sexual role as a gay man, his aesthetic role as actor and stand-up comic, and most often of his family roles as brother and son. The central focus of the session concerned his sister, Bea—their merging and his need for unconditional love.

I asked him to make up a story about a boy and a girl. The roles revealed in his many fairy-tale-like stories would provide a direct glimpse into Michael's inner world. Michael began:

> *A little boy and a little girl are alone in the house. The boy needs the girl to protect him from the monsters and the abuses of his mother. He is afraid. The source of fear is located here, in the abdomen area.*

Michael stopped speaking, paused a moment, then cried. He concluded the story with a "happily ever after" reconciliation of brother and sister. He judged the ending as unsatisfactory.

Reflecting on the story, Michael spoke of his jealousy of Bea, who always managed to have a male lover. He wanted her all for himself and fantasized about being together with her always in their loneliness. As much as he saw Bea as his double, he also recognized her power to hurt him deeply.

In Michael's story, the boy is a frightened, vulnerable victim and the girl is a powerful helper/protector. The function of the victim role is to strip power and control from an individual, making him vulnerable and helpless. The helper/protector functions to facilitate the protagonist's journey and keep him out of harm's way. As we shall see, the victim and helper roles were quite significant in Michael's search for the ring.

THE THREE BEARS

One week later, Michael brought in a letter from Bea. He had not yet read the letter, but imagined that it would say that she loved him and all was OK. He spoke with some distance about his sense of isolation in the city and his separation from Bea, who lived very far away.

I invited him to the sandtray in my office, a 4-foot by 2-foot box filled with white sand. Miniature objects, arranged by type, were on a nearby table. The categories of objects included people, nature, means of transport, animals, houses, borders, stones, and miscellaneous pieces of wood and plastic. I asked him to build a picture in the box, using as many or as few objects as he wished.

Michael built a picture with one object, a soft, small bear, which he called Barry. He said:

Barry is alone on a beach, contemplating the sand and sea. But something is missing.

He brought on a child figure, which he named Baby Blue. Barry hugs Baby Blue. They express love for one another. But something is still missing. He discovered a warrior figure and brought it into the picture. He named it Bruno.

Bruno is macho, powerful, threatening. He protects and professes love for Barry. Barry in turn protects Baby Blue.

In the end, Bruno turned away from the others. Barry's arms reached out toward him, but Bruno told him to keep his distance. Michael was then asked to disassemble the picture, placing all objects back on the table.

When we spoke about the sandplay, Michael identified Bruno as his father, and Barry and Baby Blue as roles of himself. He saw Baby Blue as the needy, childlike, vulnerable part of himself. This role allowed him to become involved in relationships, even though he generally felt alone and incapable of sustaining intimacy. He saw Barry as the maternal, protective part, but, said Michael, the feminine role was not an acceptable one. When he intoned the name, it sounded like "Bear-y."

I asked Michael whether he remembered the story "Goldilocks and the Three Bears." Michael told the story, explaining that the sandplay figures could represent the Mama Bear (Barry), the Papa Bear (Bruno), and the Baby Bear (Baby Blue). Michael then added the further character, Goldilocks, who was missing from the sandbox. The session ended.

In thinking about the session, I wondered whether Goldilocks was a version of Bea and whether the only way Michael was free to examine his relationship with his mother and father was if Bea was absent.

Three significant roles of Michael were identified during this session: Barry/Bear-y, the Mama Bear, who is maternal, protective, contemplative, and alone; Baby Blue, the Baby Bear, who is needy, childlike, and vulnerable; and Bruno, who is paternal and threatening, distant and powerful. The fourth (offstage) role of Goldilocks is most distant and poorly defined.

Taken together, these roles appeared to represent some of the dynamics of Michael's family. The father was distant and macho, and both potentially brutal and potentially protective. The mother was isolated but less distant, able to hug and thus love the child. The child was very vulnerable and suspicious of the parents, but capable of loving them at some level. The daughter/sister functioned to allow the family to address each other by virtue of being absent.

There was much potential for ambivalence in Bruno's protective power and destructive isolation, and Michael internalized the struggle between self-protection and self-destruction. I perceived a similar ambivalent quality in Barry and Baby Blue's needs for both isolation and connection.

The presentational style of Michael's drama seemed quite appropriate in identifying several major roles within his psyche. Through this style, which he would sustain throughout much of his therapy, he remained safe from his potentially overwhelming feelings of betrayal from his family. Thus he was able to highlight certain qualities of the family members, who were, after all, merely toys and bears.

THE LAWYER

In a subsequent session, Michael spoke of two relationships with men. I was not sure whether either was sexually consummated. I set up three chairs. One represented Roy, who was too underdistanced and easy to please, too vulnerable and childlike—a bit like Baby Blue. A second chair represented Paul, who lived far away. Michael described him as beautiful, distant, hard to get, and hard to keep.

I asked Michael to designate the third chair as X, whomever he wished. I suggested as examples father and ideal lover. My thinking was that Michael needed a mediator, a point of reflection or balance between the two extreme types of lovers. I thought that if he chose the father, it would be an ideal version who might serve as protector or helper. The ideal lover might offer a vision of what Michael really wanted and needed in a mate. Furthermore, in invoking these ideal types, I thought that Michael had an opportunity to explore his need for perfect figures to rescue him and make him whole. And finally, as a technical matter, I find the use of three fictional roles effective in working with a client who tends to split the world into moral polarities. The addition of the third role provides the possibility of working with alternative choices and/or within the transitional space between roles.

Michael began to take on the roles of Roy and Paul, moving in and out of their chairs. He spoke to chair X, which he identified as his ideal lover, but avoided actually taking on the role.

I asked Michael to take on the role of X directly. Noting his resistance, I asked him to close his eyes and imagine himself as X:

Who are you?

Michael.

What do you look like?

I'm wearing a suit. Clean-cut. Handsome in a conventional way.

What is your profession?

Lawyer.

What kind?

Criminal lawyer.

The lawyer went on to speak of his feelings about Michael:

> I love you, especially your sense of freedom and innocence. I am professionally and financially successful and will take care of you.

I asked Michael to tell a story about a person the lawyer defended. Michael moved quickly from the lawyer role to that of the defendant. Primarily through movement he created a man who is beaten down, hopeless, needy, but proud, refusing to seek or accept help. The defendant is a poor, homeless black man, falsely charged with robbery. Michael took on the role of the defendant with much feeling.

Four roles emerged during the session. Michael portrayed the first, Roy, as a vulnerable innocent, and the second, Paul, as a cool beauty. The third was seen by Michael as more ideal—that of the lawyer, one who is able to help and defend those who are falsely accused of crimes. Michael named the lawyer "Michael." A clear identification was thus established with this role of protector, one that Michael would continually seek out.

In reflecting upon the session, Michael said that he identified most with the defendant, the fourth role created. Michael saw himself often in this pariah role, feeling alienated from the mainstream, falsely accused of crimes that at this point had no names. During the enactment, he played out the defendant role realistically, using it to release a heavy burden of tears.

The pariah role functioned to keep Michael at bay, removed from the feared but desired world of lawyers, helpers, protectors, and successful people in suits who are able to take on adult responsibilities and love openly. If he, like his fictional defendant, refused protection, he was bound to remain oppressed, safely ensconced in his proud pariah role. Unlike his fictional counterpart, however, Michael would move on, in search of the right protection.

BLACK RAGE

Michael came into therapy exhausted and run down, worried about getting sick again. He referred to himself as unfocused and angry. I asked him to find a focus for his anger:

How does it look?

Blackness ... Rage.

A role emerged—Black Rage. Michael told a story:

Black Rage, an "it," came with my grandfather and was passed on to my father. I inherit it from my father. So does my brother and little sister. We all try to tame Black Rage through joking. But comedy fails. Black Rage has a strong hold on my father. When he acts out his Black Rage, my mother protects me. But she is ultimately powerless. The only way to get rid of Black Rage is by letting him just be. I understand this when I'm with my pregnant sister. She has a baby and we tell the baby this message. My sister, me, and the baby live happily ever after.

Following the story, I asked Michael to close his eyes and visualize a time earlier in the day when he had become angry at a bank teller who gave him a hard time cashing a check. He recognized the presence of Black Rage in his upper body—shoulders, neck, jaw. It was painful.

I asked him to re-experience the pain, then wrestle it off and throw it into the chair in front of him. He did so powerfully, then addressed Black Rage:

I want to get rid of you. Leave me alone!

I took on the role of Black Rage:

You need me. You don't really want to let me go.

We reversed roles. As Black Rage, Michael said:

The only way to let me go is through love and the letting in of real feelings.

Michael then cried openly, attempting to let go of the demon crouched on his shoulders.

Reflecting on the session, Michael mentioned that he had become aware of his mother's complicity in the cycle of anger and rage. Her part was understated and duplicitous; she worked her power from the sidelines through sarcasm and judgments. The legacy of the more direct anger was masculine, rearing its head most clearly in its descent from grandfather to father to son.

As a role type, Black Rage is a kind of demon. It appears to be born of the marriage of fear and anger. It functions to release a destructive power, frightening and threatening all those in its path. It bears some resemblance to the feminine Eumenides or Furies in Greek drama, who plague such masculine characters as the rigid, authoritarian Pentheus in *The Bacchae,* and the guilt-ridden Orestes. The legacy of Black Rage is that seen in the classical revenge tragedies and contemporary revenge films pitting blood relatives against one another.

Black Rage, as Michael conceived it, can be appeased through love and the authentic expression of feeling. But first, it must be expressed and acknowledged. As the Chorus chants in Aeschylus's *The Eumenides* (1960 ed., p. 23):

> There are times when fear is good.
> It must keep its watchful place
> at the heart's controls. There is advantage
> in the wisdom won from pain.

Perhaps the primary function of Black Rage, like that of the Furies and other dramatic demons, is to demand a place in the human psyche for that which is irrational, fearful, and rageful.

Michael's overly rational approach to negative feelings had not served him well. He was just beginning to understand the legacy of Black Rage, but was still unable to express it safely. His fear was that if he allowed himself to take on the role of Black Rage, he would become as irrational as his grandfather and father, who, as characters in his personal drama, had brutalized his psyche. Michael needed to find a style in which to express his fear and rage without feeling overwhelmed and unsafe.

At the conclusion of Aeschylus's *Orestia,* the rageful Eumenides, though defeated, are appeased by Athena and given an important moral place in the lives of Athenians. "There is advantage/in the wisdom won from pain," chants the Chorus; so, too, does wisdom spring from the expression of rage and the recognition of its place in the psyche. The search for such wisdom would provide a therapeutic goal for Michael, who left this particular session temporarily at peace, with the Black Rage in check.

THE BOY WHO LEARNED TO BURN

Michael came into therapy quite depressed. He had been sleeping most of the day, working the night shift, then going to the movies until the early morning hours. He had been thinking of the image of the house, a role left over from a previous session. For Michael, the house presented a contradiction: On the one hand, it was a safe haven, a place to eat and sleep in plenty and comfort; on the other hand, it was an unsafe representation of unloving, abusive parents.

In the previous weeks, Michael had recalled a very painful experience:

> I am young, 8 or 9, playing in the attic with some friends. I discover an old violin. I begin to play it when my father bursts into the room, clearly under the influence of the Black Rage. He yells at me, grabs the violin from my hands, and smashes it over my head. I am humiliated and in a daze. My mother is in another room, and I want her to comfort me, but she is inaccessible.

Thus, Michael saw the negative house as a place of unhappy, beaten-down children; a father who acted like an out-of-control child; and a mother who should have been a protector but appeared to be a needy child herself.

I asked Michael if he recalled his reaction to his family following the episode. He said:

> I avoided any direct confrontation. But at dinner, I remember that my father joked around a lot and everyone laughed.

I suggested that the episode still appeared to be overwhelming and that one way to approach the experience might be through humor—retelling the story as a dark comedy in order to distance himself from the powerful emotions. Michael seemed uncomfortable with this suggestion and quickly changed the subject by producing several photographs. The first one was of Michael and his siblings during Christmas. All of them appeared morose. Presents were visible, but Michael said he did not receive what he wanted. His siblings got more and better gifts. Another picture showed Michael in front of an ironing board in the dining room. He was 10.

Michael's first words in this therapy session were: "I feel foundationless." He told the story of "The Boy Who Learned to Burn":

> *Once upon a time there was a boy who liked to iron. He ironed his father's handkerchiefs and made them nice and fresh and white. He ironed his mother's things also and laid them out in two piles on the bed.*
>
> *How nice, his mother said, but his father said nothing.*
>
> *After several attempts to please his father, the boy burns his father's handkerchiefs with the iron. His father gets mad and scolds the boy and hits him. He accuses the boy of ruining his things.*
>
> *But the boy cries: I didn't do it on purpose!*

He cries and cries. (Michael cried bitterly at this point.) *He real-
izes that the only way to get his father's attention is to burn.*

Following the story, Michael spoke about the variations of burning in his own life. He was burned out and burned up. He not only
burned in the heat of the Black Rage, but easily got burned when he
was thrust into the victim role. He also tended to burn himself, to
act self-destructively, injuring his body in the process. To ease the pain
of burning, Michael withdrew into the safe narcotics of sleep, food,
and movies.

I asked Michael to look inside of the house that was himself and
tell me what he saw. Images of the living room and the fireplace came
to mind. I asked him to take on the role of the fire, and he offered
a romantic, healing picture:

I am nurturer. I warm the boy, Mikey, and make him feel good.

At the closure of the session, Michael recognized two burning
roles: that of the boy with the iron, whose uncontained, destructive
acting out demands recognition; and that of the fire, safely contained
within a fireplace, exuding healing heat and light.

The boy with the iron reflects two of Michael's role types: the
hothead and the victim. Trapped in a house with a violent, uncaring
father, Michael could only hope to get attention through acting out
provocatively. In the story, the hotheaded boy with the iron serves
this purpose well. The burning of his father's handkerchiefs represents
Michael's futile cries to be seen by his father. As victim, the boy gets
what he wants—the father's attention. But instead of the desired love
from his father, the boy gets the Black Rage.

The mother role remains, for the most part, undeveloped. She
is pleased by the boy's handiwork, and thus removed from his hurt
and consequent anger.

The role of the fire, an abstraction, functioned to move Michael
along his journey toward reconstructing a psychologically safe house
to live in. Fire is paradoxical in its potential for destruction, as in the
hands of an angry victim with a hot iron, and domesticity, as in its
containment within a fireplace. Michael, like many angry men and
women, was searching for the contained hearth that would support
his wounded heart.

FATHERS AND SONS

Michael was cast in a new play set in the South. He played Bo, a
12-year-old boy—innocent, moral, and fondly attached to his older

sister, who is his constant companion throughout the play. He is the narrator, telling the story of his father, Julian, a lawyer who defends a black man falsely accused of a crime. Bo has great respect for his father, a moral model who loves his son. I wondered whether it was coincidental that the roles of lawyer and defendant, a falsely accused black man, were repeated in Michael's life.

Michael came into therapy speaking in a Southern accent. He explained that the accent was essential for his character and he needed to practice it all the time, but he also expressed some doubt:

> I am afraid you won't approve.
>
> Why?
>
> Because it keeps me from my real feelings.

I asked Michael to take on the role of Bo. He did so:

> I don't get enough of my father. I'm lost. I would like to meet someone to take care of me. I would like to go away to a Spanish speaking country and teach Spanish to the children. (*He corrected himself:*) English, I mean.

After de-roling, Michael relaxed. He spoke normally—no more accent. We spoke about the best ways to play a character, keeping a balance between actor and role. When an actor is too submerged in the role, there is no room to reflect, to alter, to make sense of the enactment.

Michael then spoke about a significant episode in his nontheatrical life. He had returned home for Christmas and decided to finally confront his father for his humiliations and abuses. Without guilt, the father replied:

> But I was just a child myself. I'm still a child and will always be a child. You can't expect me to be different.

Initially, Michael was relieved. But then the sadness set in, followed by depression:

> How can I get my needs met from a child? I need a father. I need apologies. I need to forgive him. How can I do this if he is just like me?

The two prominent roles here were father and son. In Michael's real-life drama, the function of the son was to attempt to elicit the approval, apology, and love from the father. The function of the father was to withhold the desired apologies and to challenge the son to take care of himself.

In this session the roles of father and son coexisted on three different levels: the theatrical level of Bo and Julian; the therapeutic level of client and therapist; and the everyday level of Michael and his father.

The qualities of both roles can be compared on all three levels. Bo would appear to be the least needy child, with a clearly defined father/moral model worthy of his love. Yet, as portrayed in the therapy session by Michael, he needs more of his father's time and attention. His father doesn't take care of him enough. He needs to take on the father role himself in a foreign land and teach the children how to speak their own language—that is, how to make sense of their own lives and communicate with others. Julian, the father, is adult, loving, moral, powerful, yet somewhat aloof. His primary concern is his professional role.

Michael, the client, was also respectful of the adult father figure, the therapist. He needed my approval for being a good actor and a good Bo. Yet he thought that I would only fully approve if he was able, first, to resist a merging with the Bo role, and second, to use the Bo role to get to an authentic level of feeling. Thus, my approval was conditional, dependent upon his competence as a therapeutic role player. The quality of my role as a drama therapist, as Michael saw it, was consistent—like Julian, adult, caring, professional, yet also somewhat aloof.

Michael as son to his father was most needy. Not only did he need his father's time and attention, but also his forgiveness and approval. The father was the least accepting of the three adult figures. In the past, he had transformed the son into a victim to his Black Rage. When accused by the son later, the father constructed the perfect alibi—not guilty by reason of childishness.

There were other levels upon which the father–son transference appeared in Michael's theatrical life. It would be played out in his stormy relationship to the director of the play, a highly temperamental, childish, passive–aggressive type who would alienate his cast and be forced to close down the run of the show prematurely; and to the actor playing Julian, a kindly gentleman who openly praised Michael's performance.

The father–son motif is a mainstay of drama. It is the struggle between Oedipus and Laius, Abraham and Isaac, Hamlet and Claudius, Christy Mahon and his Old Mahon in *The Playboy of the Western World,* Jamie and James Tyrone in *Long Day's Journey into Night,* Biff and Willy Loman in *Death of a Salesman.* The dramatic struggle, epitomized by Freud in his psychological musings on the drama of Oedipus, has been extended by Jones (1949/1976) into the psychic domicile of Hamlet.

The ultimate goal of the son, exemplified well by Michael, is to move beyond the attachment to the mother and resentment toward the father, transferring his love to an appropriate, nonincestuous mate. The role of the son often takes on heroic proportions as he journeys toward acquiring the power, wisdom, blessing, and identity of the father.

The father role becomes more diverse in its symbolic association with God and with many kinds of male authority figures (e.g., directors, therapists, teachers, warriors). The father role easily becomes an abstraction, an ideal, and then, more realistically, a disappointment. When Michael discovered that his father, whose approval he needed so desperately, was no more than a son, himself a child, he was confused and depressed. How could he search for someone who had no more power and authority than himself? Michael was not prepared to recognize this type of father. But if a father is like a son, then the son has the power to grant himself the things he has always needed from the father. This thought was not yet available to Michael; for me, however, it served as a touchstone.

THE JUDGE AND THE RAINCOAT

In the play Michael was rehearsing, the character, Bo, dominates the first act but has little to do in the second act. The director asked Michael to double up and play a small role, that of the Judge. He was resistant, angry.

In therapy, Michael took on the Judge role. I asked him to speak in character about his occupation and the functions he serves. He did so:

> The first function is to criticize. The second is to support and protect.
>
> How do you protect?
>
> Well, for one thing, I remind you to wear a raincoat. And one more thing—I also overprotect. This makes you feel lost, insignificant, invisible.

When I asked Michael to name the Judge, he offered "Justin." He had no conscious associations with that name. Could it be an abbreviation of justice, the moral principle that influenced his search for a good father? Could it be an incomplete phrase, as in "just in time"? Just in time for what? Perhaps from being sentenced to a life of alienation and insignificance, one in which the possibility of moral justice has vanished?

Toward the end of the session, Michael recounted an actual incident:

> I was restless last night and couldn't sleep. I called the sex line and was invited to this guy's house who happened to live in the neighborhood. To protect myself, I went in the role of Bo, the Southern boy. I wanted to be in control. Bo called the shots. The sex was safe and enjoyable: masturbating, no touching. The other guy wanted to go further and demanded more. As Michael, I might have had trouble resisting, but Bo didn't. He said no and left.

The role worked. Michael had fun and met his needs even as he took control. The critical and overprotective judges were silenced. The protective Judge was active and in consort with Bo, allowing safe sex and safe feeling.

The image of the raincoat came up at this point. On the one hand, it related to safe sex, a kind of somatic prophylactic; on the other hand, it took on a more psychological significance. Michael recalled an old photograph. He was a young boy in a raincoat, sitting outside the house, but it wasn't raining out. As we spoke about the image, Michael became aware of his need to find a way to link the appropriate protection with the appropriate role. Why play the role of one who needs protection when there is no danger? Why wear a raincoat when it is not raining?

If the Judge is the protector who "reminds you to wear a raincoat," then one needs to know when to call him forth in order to feel protected. Michael needed to let go of the two other functions of the Judge in order for the protective function to emerge fully. The critic is the enemy of the searcher, exposing and slowing him down, inducing guilt and self-doubt rather than helping him move ahead on his journey. The overprotector is also a heavy burden, falsely calling himself a helper but actually functioning to deprive the searcher of his independence.

When he finally assumed the Judge role in the play, Michael's resistance and anger were gone. The Judge of Act II did not at all overshadow or demean Bo of Act I. If anything, Michael learned how to integrate the two. And life reflected art, in that Michael also recognized that by integrating the roles of innocent and protector he could even enjoy anonymous sex, which in the past he had bitterly criticized and regretted.

A more significant integration yet to come, I thought, was how the protective judge could lead the vulnerable, hurt Michael further along the way toward assuming the father role himself—moving from child to adult, from victim to hero.

THE MASK OF THE ACTOR

The play opened. Michael paced himself, saving his best emotional stuff for the second weekend, when his family came to the theatre. On the day of his father's 60th birthday, they arrived—father, mother, brother, and family friends. They adored Michael's performance. Michael joined the family for dinner following the performance; he ate abundantly. At midnight, they all sang "Happy Birthday" to his father. Michael was glad to join in.

Although there were several weeks left to the run, Michael felt depressed and empty. He had a dream:

> I take my makeup off after a performance and I'm in San Francisco. I'm lost, lonely.

Underneath the persona of the performer is a lost person, a stranger. In quality, the performer role is like a narcotic—addictive and capable of blocking out the pull and responsibilities of other roles. It offers a momentary fix, but leaves an emptiness behind, a desire for more. The performer role helps one distance from the reality of the everyday.

Within Michael's imagination, the performer role spawned the subroles of Bo and the Judge, both of which served him well. Bo, who is respectful and loving of his father and attached to his sister, functioned as a representation of Michael's ideal relationship to his father and sister. The role of Bo also provided a goal for Michael. I asked him:

> What do you think will become of Bo when he grows up.

> I am not sure of his sexuality, but I think he will be a lawyer like his father.

Bo's goal, then, as Michael saw it, is to become a defender and protector, a model and moral father for other sons.

In many ways, however, the performer role had become too dominant within Michael's personality. His dream might well be saying: Take away the theatrical personae and the person, Michael, is lost, like one of Pirandello's six characters in perpetual search of an author.

In a subsequent session, Michael spoke further of the actor/performer role.

> While onstage I worry about being seen. I'm afraid of stealing a scene, drawing too much attention to myself. On the other hand, I'm more concerned about being ignored, of not being seen enough.

> This is an actor's fundamental dilemma, I thought—to be seen or not to be seen.

A primary function of the performer role is to communicate a feeling or idea through a character. To communicate effectively, actors must assert themselves through the role, drawing forth a reaction from the audience. At the most basic level, that reaction is based upon an acceptance of an actor in role. The function of the audience is to accept the dramatic reality of the actors as characters, responding to them not as persons but as personae. In Michael, whose issues concerned an underdeveloped role system and an overdependence upon judges, fathers, and other critical audiences, the invalidation of a role equaled an invalidation of the one acting the role. If Bo/Judge was unseen, so was Michael. A primary reason why Michael acted was to achieve validation. And to get it, he needed to find a way to play his performer role that was not either too demanding of the audience (drawing too much attention to himself) or too removed from the audience (fading into the scenery).

So, too, did Michael struggle with his need to be seen by his family and peers. When acting most childlike, he exhibited himself presentationally—becoming the stand-up comic who made people laugh but remained distant, or the little innocent boy who either withdrew to the seashore to commune with nature, or opened himself up too much to hurt, exposing his vulnerability. When acting most adult, Michael took on a more representational style—endowing his roles with feeling, attempting to be seen.

Michael began to speak of an entirely new subrole of the performer: that of the businessman, the entrepreneur, one who must look after his own interests, organize pictures and resumes, procure an agent and paying work. To be seen as an actor on stage or in everyday life, reasoned Michael, one must be allowed to act. The businessman role provides that by moving the actor closer to a professional goal, and by offering assistance (in the form of pictures, resumes, and theatrical agents) to insure that the actor will get there.

THE CRITIC

I was about to leave for a sabbatical trip to Europe. Closure of this phase of therapy was drawing near. Michael had a dream:

> I know you've written a review of me as Bo, and I pick up the review, but I can't find the parts you've written.

I asked him to visualize the review and find the missing part. He read it:

> Michael is energetic, wonderful, the best thing in the play.

Michael began to speak openly about me for the first time:

A few weeks ago I began to see you as imperfect. You misunder-
stood the meaning of the violin episode. I thought it was pretty
stupid to suggest humor as a solution to my humiliation. Before
that time, you were an ideal to me—like a good father. But you
disappointed me, and I punished you by cutting off my feelings
in therapy. My experiences in theatre became a substitute.

By finding the positive review in his imagination, Michael was
able to reassert a positive transference. I did not become an ideal father,
like the character Julian, fixed by his fictional presence in a given text.
Rather, I became more real both for failing him and for standing by
him uncritically. Although as therapist I was less than ideal, as review-
er/critic I was reliable, capable of offering positive judgment. Perhaps,
however, Michael saw that judgment as too positive.

It may have been that the thought of my leaving necessitated my
transformation into the ideal, uncritical critic. In many ways, roles
were still very moral for Michael. Like Bo, Michael needed justice and
needed a father to defend him against the injustices of the world.
Michael also needed to judge and punish his father for his abuses
and his inability to assume an adult role. Furthermore, Michael needed
to assume a lawyer role himself, and became cognizant of the fact
that when one fights the good battle, as the character Julian does,
goodness and justice do not always prevail. Finally, he needed to accept the thought that it is in the fight itself where meaning resides.

THE BLIND GIRL

The play closed prematurely. I was about to leave on sabbatical.
Michael was about to take a trip out West. There were many closures
at hand. Michael brought in a figure in a dream, Patty. In quality, she
was the other side of the energetic, innocent Baby Blue. Patty was
hollow-eyed, depressed, beaten down. She is blind and mute, overdistanced and passive.

I asked Michael to visualize Patty. Although he expected me to
ask him to take on the role of Patty, I shifted and asked him to play
himself in relation to Patty. He made the shift easily and began to
stroke the air. He spoke to Patty: "It's all right." He was a father holding his baby. I took off my sweater, bunched it up, and gave it to him.
Michael held the object tenderly and said: Don't cry, Patty. He comforted, assured and protected her.

Two roles were powerfully present in Michael's portrayal. The first was the victim as abused, silenced child, who is the object of the Black Rage. The second was the protector as nurturing father, mature adult, protective judge—one who loves uncritically, even if the love object is imperfect.

Michael's style of enactment was balanced, evoking deep feeling as well as reflection. After crying, he said:

> I feel a great sense of relief and clarity. I know Patty very well. She lives inside me.

I found myself full of feeling as never before with Michael. The image of the ring came to mind. Was this the connection, the bond that could finally be dramatized directly, with father and child playing out their appropriate roles—the father as strong, dependable, loving; the child as dependent, imperfect, vulnerable?

We talked about the meaning of the roles and the tasks that remained: for the adult/father role to contain that of the wounded child; and for the child/victim to allow herself to be seen by the adult/father; and for the victim/abused child role to have less control and power over the entire system of roles that was Michael's personality.

AN INTEGRATION

In the last session before I left, Michael reported another dream:

> The central figure is Billy, a young, fat boy. Billy tells his mother that he wants to be left alone. His mother argues with him. As an adult, I take Billy's side against the mother. But Billy turns to me and tells me, quite firmly, that I must also leave him alone. Billy says: "I can fight my own battles!"

The overweight quality of Billy seemed significant. I asked Michael whether he knew the Franz Kafka story "A Hunger Artist" (1924/1952). He didn't, and I told him the story this way:

> A man whose art is fasting is asked why he continues to fast, even after his audiences have long since abandoned him. He replies, "Because I could never find the right food."
>
> But Billy is different, Michael responded. He found the right emotional food. In confronting the world of adults and taking an independent stand, he feeds himself.

The image of the fat boy was a powerful one for Michael who, in fact, always stuffed himself with food provided by his parents when visiting home, but never gained weight.

We spoke of the possibility of integrating a number of significant roles: Billy, Patty, Bo, Baby Blue. We spoke of these being all
children—the internalized child role, split into many parts. Michael
described the qualities and functions of each, and I commented on
his descriptions:

> Patty is like a cannonball who gets what she wants by rolling her-
> self up and throwing herself into a crowd.

> The role of victim functions destructively and masochistically,
> like the boy who learned to burn.

> Baby Blue kills by loving people to death and manipulating them
> into loving him.

> The role of innocent can serve a manipulative function. This, too,
> is a destructive path that ultimately wounds the innocent.

> Billy and Bo know the right foods to eat.

> Both are forms of child heroes—the former independent and emo-
> tionally satiated; the latter moral, respectful, and loving. Both
> search for a way to be fathered. Bo's way is to emulate a positive
> model; Billy's way is to steer clear of a negative one. Both are
> desperately needed.

We were concluding 1 year of drama therapy. The major child
role types were now visible and nameable: the innocent, Baby Blue;
the idealist, Bo; the victim, Patty; the warrior, Billy. In the identification of these roles, Michael came to see certain parts of himself that
were not clear before. In working through the roles he was attempting to find a balance among them, so that any one would not usurp
too much power from his role system. That balance would come not
only through the child roles, but also through those of Julian (the
lawyer), Judge, Black Rage, and other father roles and feminine roles
already discovered but yet to be integrated.

Before we closed, Michael addressed me directly for the second
time, pointing out the difficulties he had in opening up to me when
I remained closed, entrenched in my therapist role. He acknowledged
my power to hurt him.

I had become very human to him, both therapist and father, both
accepting critic and critical judge. I could now be addressed directly
and looked in the eyes. I had seen him, even though I had not allowed him to see me. His function and mine differed, and this was
OK. In fact, it was something he wanted very much in his relationship with his father—a separation, a tacit acceptance of each other's
roles. Lacking this, drama therapy became a positive substitute, in
many ways an alternative model of father and son.

With the acknowledgment of more work to be done, of searching for ways to lead Billy and Bo into adulthood and to further diffuse the power of Patty and the Black Rage, we agreed to resume our work after 4 months' time. For the first time in a year, we shook hands. I put my hand on his shoulder, somewhat tentatively. We were both uncomfortable. But the attempt was made, the difficult touch of therapist and client, father and son, man and man.

CHAPTER FIVE

The Case of Michael:
Part II

THE KISS

After a 4-month break, Michael resumed drama therapy. He began by talking rapidly about a love affair that had gone nowhere, about purchasing his first grown-up bed, a single. I asked:

Why a single?

My room was small. I have back problems. It's all I could afford, anyway.

I wondered, silently, whether the single bed was a way of maintaining his adolescent role. I wondered whether Michael was now in an adolescent phase and how powerfully the child roles would figure in his therapy.

He looked different. He had grown a goatee and mustache, which made him look older, more sophisticated.

The goatee helps me play my masculine role.

How are things with your father?

OK.

He proceeded to speak about his mother. She was hyper, childlike. She needed to be needed. He wanted to help her.

She was like my little sister.

I asked Michael to take on the role of the mother. He started to speak, but stammered. His body was tense. He got up and moved around the room, more fluid now. Steve, her older son, was about to be married.

I can't do anything. It's out of my hands. They've taken care of everything. There's nothing for me to do. It's all out of my control. It's very frustrating, my son's wedding and I have nothing to do.

Michael de-roled and spoke:

Steve was marrying our mother. She'll smother him, make him feel needed, but will keep him dependent and infantile. . . . My mother is a little girl. She feels ugly, no purpose, unseen. Her sister was beautiful. She wasn't. She's so needy, so alone.

How are you like your mother?

I need to be needed. When I play the feminine role I feel unsafe. But I want to play it. I am a needy child, a neglected child, like Patty.

Although there was no evidence that his mother was abused, Michael made a connection between the mother and Patty. In Michael's eyes the mother often behaved as if she were abused, blind, and totally vulnerable. Michael's identification with both female characters was strong.

Before the wedding, Michael went on a camping trip with Steve, needing to be alone with him. Michael acknowledged that Steve was like their father in many ways. While camping, they had fun laughing together and singing obscene songs. Michael reflected:

I was in my feminine energy. Maybe other people thought we were a gay couple.

I asked Michael how he became gay. Was it a choice? He was upset by the suggestion of a choice:

Who would choose to be gay? I always liked to play the feminine roles. I don't remember when I became aware of being attracted to men, but they were always the ones that made me excited.

In a dream, Michael had made love to a woman and enjoyed it. He spoke of a close woman friend with whom he had "messed around," playing sexually, no penetration, nothing unsafe. He also told of his sister Bea barging in on him when he was 12 and naked in the bathtub. She told him that Steve came into her room at night and masturbated. Michael was ashamed of his nakedness and told her, angrily:

I can't do anything about it! Why ask me what to do?

He felt guilty about his inability to offer help, but reasoned that, after all, he was just a kid when this happened. I wondered whether he was still using this rationalization in his sexual encounters.

Michael told me of a recent sexual experience:

> I met an older man who invited me to his apartment and began to seduce me. I expected more—a relationship, at least being seen. But I was a sexual object, and part of me liked that. The older man penetrated me. I got very angry and pulled away. The man fell asleep and I left. I beat myself up for days.

More sexual memories poured out:

> As a young adolescent, I was under Bea's bed. Steve was also there. We were all supposed to masturbate. I had an orgasm, but was dry. I saw the wet on Steve and felt confused.

I recalled Michael's story of being a young boy in his parent's bed, his father on the floor, naked, doing push-ups—Michael trying hard not to look but wanting so much to see.

Michael met a young man on the street. They didn't become lovers, but they held each other, clothed, kidding rather than kissing. I thought Michael said "hitting." He explained that a kiss from his father was sometimes like a hit, or that the family's kiss was a kid, a joke, a defense against feeling. The kiss as a tender expression of love was absent from the family and absent from Michael's sex life.

The sexual dynamics of Michael's family were beginning to surface, with hints of incest and further evidence of role ambivalence. Michael was trying very hard to portray a masculine role: He grew hair on his face, he played big brother to his mother's little sister; he went camping with his older brother. But his confusions surfaced in a flurry of incestuous images. Steve, the older brother, became an Oedipal character in marrying his mother. He and Steve might have been secret lovers in a tent. Could the female lover in his dream have been his mother or sister? He was drawn into a web of incestuous play by his brother and sister. Finally, he was seduced and feminized by an older man who may well have been a persona of the father.

To sort this all out, Michael needed to be reminded of the prototypical role qualities and functions of the father, mother, brother, sister, and lover. The kiss of each type has a different meaning. The parents' and siblings' kiss should be loving in a safe and nonsexual way. The lover's kiss can be more complex—sometimes the kid, sometimes the hit, sometimes the seduction, sometimes the safe and loving embrace of a peer from a distinctly different bloodline.

THE WOODEN CLOGS AND THE RUBBER BOOTS

Michael suspected that there was some connection between his sexuality and the humiliations he suffered at the hands of his father. He told a story:

There was a little boy who sings and goes with girls and stares at the ocean. His father was a fisherman. He smells of fish. He has shining eyes. The boy wears clogs. The father wears rubber boots. The boy walks down the cobblestone street toward the father, but the father thinks it's a girl.

When are you going to become a man and wear rubber boots? says the Father.

I like my clogs.

Women wear clogs.

The boy was in the shower, his clogs on the floor. The father comes in and sees the clogs and was angry. He chops them up with an ax. The boy comes out and sees his father laughing.

I've made you a man. I've cut up your clogs.

They were mine! The boy was furious.

If you want to be a woman I will chop off your penis with my ax, says the father.

The boy runs to his mother: Daddy's trying to make me into a woman

He's just kidding. It's all right, son.

The father buys a pair of rubber boots for his son. They fit well. He gives his son a big hug and tells him he loves him.

Go away, I hate you

Everyone who sees the boy tells him how well he looks and that now he was a man. But the boy goes to the sea and throws away the boots, and forever after he walks around barefoot

The moral of the story was: No one can tell you who you are by the shoes you wear on your feet

In this story, Michael highlighted the central issues concerning the father and son roles. The father as sexual model and authority must impose his masculine legacy upon his son, laying his sexuality at his feet. The son/novice was mistrustful for good reason. He was not permitted any choice in the matter. His sexual difference, expressed by his choice of shoes, was not taken into consideration. He must submit to the overbearing sexual authority of the father or become brutally stripped of his masculinity. The son's function was thus to resist malevolent male authority that can humiliate and emasculate.

The son sees the mother role as a potential helper and ally, if not a savior. Yet the mother abrogates those motherly qualities, choosing denial rather than nurturance. Her purpose, then, was to further the son's frustration, anger, and fear. From Michael's point of view, both parents refuse to play out their expected role functions. Consequently, as son he was lost.

The story takes an odd turn when the father further manipulates the boy through feigning love, and the people of the town, a kind of chorus, affirm the father's point of view. In the conventional masculine role, the boy looks good. If the shoes fit, they seem to say to the son, then wear them. Take on the role of the father and all will be well.

This part of the story reveals Michael's sexual ambivalence. If only he were acceptable to the people! If only he could step into his father's boots and smell and look like a man! Yet, in doing so, he would be cutting off a major part of himself—the homosexual part and the part needing to integrate the masculine with the feminine. The ambivalence was too overwhelming for the boy. His resolution, like the moral of the story, was unsatisfactory: He chooses not to be sexual, hoping to become invisible. The role of the barefoot boy was that of the pariah—in this case, a sexual outcast, one who has not made up his mind as to who he was as a sexual being.

Michael needed to find the right shoes, the right sexual role that would integrate the boy and the man, the masculine and the feminine, the gentle and the brutal. Once the sexual ambiguities were recognized and taken on, then a chorus would be less necessary to tell Michael who he was. In his father's terrible sexuality lay the seeds of Michael's liberation—not into the trade of fishing, but shoemaking.

Michael told of another real-life version of a sexual father–son relationship. Michael and an older man spoke to each other on a telephone sex line with some regularity. They referred to each other with endearments of the father-and-son variety, all of which led to erotic sex talk and masturbation. Michael was afraid to meet this man in person, afraid that he would be too old and unattractive. Perhaps his greatest fear was an incestuous one—the ultimate ambiguity. Yet again, Michael recalled the scene in his parent's bed, watching television cuddled up to his mother as his father performed his macho ritual on the floor. The ambivalent boy wanted so much to look, but dared not. What would he see? The size of the sexual father role was as terrifying then to the young boy as it was now to the young adult.

THE MARRIAGE PROPOSAL

Michael was playing the role of Lomov, a weak, frazzled, complaining hypochondriac, in Chekhov's *The Marriage Proposal* (1935). He complained that the role wasn't working for him. He could not find the humor. He was becoming tired of acting.

When I asked Michael what function Lomov serves in the play, he responded:

To get someone to take care of him.

That statement proved quite relevant to his real-life condition; failing to get his needs met by his parents, he looked for them in his sister and various lovers.

We spoke of the style of presentation of Lomov. Michael saw him as overstated, funny, and ridiculous, compulsive and rigid. He was emblematic of one cut off from his feelings, overdistanced, in need of the regulated life. I asked Michael how these qualities related to his own life:

I don't like to acknowledge this part of me. I also want to be the traveler, free-spirited, unregulated. Can I be this?

I asked Michael to take on the role of Lomov, staying with the presentational style, playing him larger than life:

I'm cold. I'll catch cold. I'll lie in bed and not be able to do anything. My leg hurts. I can't go riding. Ohhhh. (*He held his neck.*) I need someone to take care of me. I'm so broken up. Nobody cares I'm so hurt. I can have a heart attack at any moment. I need some stupid woman to take care of me so I don't have to deal with getting up any more. I have to go to the doctor to get more pills.

Michael's enactment was realistic; it came from his Method training and attempts to avoid cliché. It wasn't funny or ridiculous at all, but claustrophobic. I asked Michael to place Lomov in an empty chair and comment upon his enactment. In the critic role, Michael commented:

You're constantly complaining. You're a mass of insecurities held up in your body. Nobody's going to take care of you. You're all twisted up. How did that happen? I feel angry at you. You have a choice to let it all go or live with it. I don't believe all your ailments. You're just trying to get someone to take care of you. Why don't you do it yourself?

The role of Lomov was a familiar one to Michael, and he recognized that after the commentary. His inability to play the fictional Lomov, he noted, was related to his frustration with the Lomov part of himself in real life—the whiny, passive, hypochondriac who was unable to become the butt of his own ridicule. He needed distance. I advised him to temper his Method training with more style, to use the role as a way of making fun of himself when he was like Lomov.

He was reminded of the function of humor in his family. It was a weapon forcing him into a victim role. His mother used it expertly to ridicule him and his siblings. He again referred to this form of negative humor as "hitting." An alternative form of good humor, according to Michael, involved playful, childish kidding that served a healing purpose. He liked to play and kid with his siblings.

We spoke of ways in which Michael could play the ridiculous quality of Lomov without feeling the sting of his mother's brand of humor. We then spoke of the function of the Lomov role, which Michael recognized as pointing out to an audience the silliness that comes from self-pity. Through the humor of the character, the audience should be able to laugh at those qualities of themselves. And Michael would then be able to laugh with them. He, too, could transcend his self-piteous, egocentric, victim role through laughter, which in itself offers a way to deal with ambiguity.

The hurting–healing ambiguity in laughter would be manageable if Michael could rediscover the joy in acting. He left the session with this thought:

> If I can have fun again, then I can again breathe life into my roles. This is what it's all about.

It was also about putting the pieces of the personality back together again, I thought—a Humpty-Dumpty-type job, larger than the efforts of all the king's horses and all the king's men.

THE GLASS HEART

Once upon a time, a little boy and a little girl played in the sun. They sang and were carefree. The boy spotted the dark Prince. He wanted the Prince to put him on a horse and ride him around town. Instead, the Prince picked up the girl. The boy was crushed. The mother and the father watched and told the boy to be happy because the Prince picked up the girl.

Years went by. The Prince picked up the girl again and again. The boy noticed that she was wearing a glass heart She told him that the Prince gave it to her.

The boy was about to go far away. The girl said:

Don't leave me. I'm afraid.

I'm afraid, too.

You must remember me. Here, take this heart Always keep it with you.

The little boy sailed away and held the heart and felt good. Part of him felt bad because the heart was from the Prince. One day, in a war, a sword hit the boy and he got sick. In the hospital he noticed that the heart was gone. He wished that he had died.

He went back to the war and forgot about the heart, the Prince, and the sister. After the war, he went home. The town was destroyed. All was gone. He sailed to a faraway isle. In a cave he found a piece of glass shaped like a heart. He cut his hair, entwined it around the glass heart, and tied it around his neck. He now had his sister's love and all the love around him.

I asked Michael to speak from the point of view of all the characters. He first spoke as the Prince:

> I have fought long and hard. I want some place to sit down, to raise my family. The war was ending but it still goes on. I'm searching for that home.

As the little girl, he said:

> I have love, beauty. I have lost my people but I still have my heart. I can continue to love and forgive because that was what I was born for.

As the heart, Michael said:

> I am the healing stone, the representation of the human condition. I have the power to keep people together. I am a balancer, feminine and masculine, boy and girl. I am the greatest gift of all.

Finally, I asked Michael to play the boy. He replied:

> I did. I played the boy grown up. That was my first speech.
>
> I thought you played the Prince.

Michael was confused. The role of the little boy had merged with that of the Prince. When he was able to make the separation, he took on the role of the little boy:

> I love the shining Prince I saw. I want him to love me for who I am. But I see that I am not lovable because she was more lovable to him. I am alone. I have a heart so big in me. My parents watch me as my heart is breaking. They tell me not to cry, that I should be happy for her. But I have a heart of glass and it might shatter forever.

As the heart, he continued:

> I am the heart. I am born again in the little boy. I am your heart now. You can be loved again even if you are not her. The love comes from me, not from the Prince. I am your heart and you will be loved.

Michael spoke of the image of the glass heart. He had just turned 28 years old. He needed to allow the feminine role to come out and be seen. As a birthday present to himself, he bought a glass heart. But on his way to therapy, a homophobic man saw how he was dressed and ridiculed him.

In the wars outside, through the abuse and neglect of the symbolic fathers and mothers, through their constant refusal to take on the savior role, Michael easily lost heart. The same wars raged inside Michael.

In the story the role of the heart was resurrected, discovered in a cave, a recess within Michael's psyche. The heart serves well as a transitional object standing between the feminine and masculine parts of Michael. In telling he story, he described it as a gift. And as a gift it becomes the healing role, vulnerable and transparent as glass, but resilient and transformative. The heart has the potential power to allow the feminine role to surface, to allow the Prince part of the boy to assert adult masculine power, to link the two sexual roles, and to transform the rejected boy into one who is lovable. Michael had trouble taking on the Prince role, because his own adult masculine power was still too underdeveloped and frightening.

The heart is a complex role. Its origins are in both the Prince, a betrayer, and the sister, a lover. It highlights Michael's ambivalence of love and betrayal, along with those of safe sex and incest and of masculine and feminine identities. The fairy-tale style of presentation helped Michael explore that ambivalence by highlighting the moral issues and distancing him from an emotional overload.

The Prince was a representation of the father, a figure that was sometimes terrifying, often confusing. Like the Prince in the story, the father figure saves and betrays and passes on his male legacy through the female. In the absence of positive male models, Michael looked to the women in his family and found further confusions, seeing his mother and sister as masculine women in demeanor and attitude.

In his struggle, Michael looked to the possibilities of sexual integration, of liberating the feminine part of himself, without fearing the loss of the masculine. Even though he had not yet found the right shoes, perhaps by wearing the glass heart he might move closer toward that "fearful symmetry" (see Blake, "The Tyger" [1794/1960]).

BUGS

Michael was supposed to be the final child in the family. His mother wanted a girl. It was a difficult, painful birth. His mother and father tried to kill the pain through humor. Michael said:

They tried real hard to get me. My mother feared a daughter but she wanted a daughter. She was late. The labor was induced. She became real giddy in the final stages, and when I was born, my mother laughed me out. Since I can remember, she has always referred to me as "Mama's boy."

When the parents tried again for a girl, Bea was born. Soon thereafter, Michael began seeing bugs. When Bea was first in the presence of a doctor, Michael said:

I saw Bea as a spider.

Michael had a terror of bugs. He recalled an early incident when he was sick with a high fever. He went to the bathroom, half delirious. A large water bug crossed his bare foot. He was terrified.

Michael had taken on a new lover, Joe, a young, very attractive man he met in the park. Although afraid of the sex, Michael allowed himself to relax and assumed a feminine sexual role. This felt unsatisfactory. I asked:

Who taught you that it was bad to be feminine?

Not my father. I think my mother. Sex was so strange in our family. I think Bea was attracted to me sexually. When Bea was small, Steve would come into her room and mess around.

If you could have a solid, mature relationship with Joe, what would you be willing to give up?

My parents. Everything. Never see them again.

But then Michael's critical side appeared:

But Joe is too humorless. He is not one of the family.

The ambivalence intensified. Michael would give up his family for his lover, but unless his lover were one of the family, he would give up his lover. In fact, many of the ambivalences became Michael's fears, his bugs.

MORE GLASS

Michael recalled a dream:

There was a limp gun, a kid's gun, like a cap gun. It needs ammunition. I try to force the wrong ammo in to get a bang. Bea gave me the ammo. I need to fire it at the glass. I fire. The glass doesn't break. But the shot leaves a brown mark on the glass.

Michael was very agitated. Joe had rejected him. He tried so hard to meet men, and they all rejected him. He was the victim and was very angry. There was a piano in the room, and I asked him to play. He found sharply contrasting sounds—a persistent, heavy bass and a fluttering treble. There were few middle tones. Afterward, he spoke of the contrast and the need to find a middle range.

I asked Michael to translate each musical register into a role, one already defined. The low tones became the Black Rage, the high ones Glass. I asked him to use sound and movement to invoke both roles, and to move from one to another at will.

As Black Rage, Michael began to punch out. His arms flailed like a windmill. He hit the air with power. He uttered guttural and retching sounds. As Glass, he reached out with open arms. His sounds were stifled cries. He ended up rolling on the floor and sobbing, then came to rest, exhausted:

I feel good. The rage is gone.

We spoke of ways to temper the Black Rage, to let it go through acknowledging the hurt and expressing it in some appropriate way. The sexual ambivalence was again present: The Glass was feminine, too vulnerable, capable of breaking at any moment; the Black Rage masculine, too overpowering.

Michael's dream indicates his great continuing need to be like his father, the conventional male—macho, strong, sexual, carrying a deadly gun with real bullets. Yet his gun in the dream is limp and depleted of male energy. Only a girl can give him his potency, and even then it is not the right stuff. As for the glass, it is too transparent, only capable of deflecting a weak attempt at potency. Michael thus continued his search for the elusive balance, the ability to live in his ambivalence and hold the parts together.

MI VIDA ABAJO (MY LIFE DOWN THERE)

It was fall and the weather was turning cold. The people of the city were coming down with the flu. Michael needed to protect himself from the flu bugs and stay healthy. He told me that he had, in the past, tested positive for a number of viruses, including an odd one that only pregnant women get. He said:

Maybe I can fight off the AIDS virus, too. I would never take AZT if I had AIDS because I don't want any toxic things in my body.

The night before, Michael had discovered a giant water bug in his kitchen.

I was afraid, terrified, but I chased it down, knocking over everything in the kitchen, and I killed it. It was a war zone in there. Amazing, but I slept through the night.

The warrior role of Michael was surfacing, and as it did, the victim role was losing some of its power. He was beginning to discover that in mobilizing the strength to kill the demonic water bugs that ran around his house like harpies, he was preparing for a more frightening showdown with the interior bugs of doubt, fear, and rage.

Often, his life narrative jumped from the representational stories of bugs in the kitchen to the more romantic, escapist kind, such as the following:

A young gay actor, who knew he had greatness in him but knew that he couldn't always be great, wanted to see other cultures and hear other voices. He wanted to go where there was warmth in the winter and smiles and oceans. So he flew out of the exhaust and noise of the cold city and landed in a beautiful green haven. The people were warm and accepted him for what he was. In town there was a serenity and peace, and he wrote down his thoughts in Spanish. He met many beautiful men, who were attracted to him for his blue eyes and different coloration. With one Spanish-speaking man in particular, he spent days and nights together on the beach. They held hands and took long walks. There was nothing more that he wanted. Then it was time to get back on the plane. He looked into the black eyes of his lover:

I have to leave now.
You must stay.
I need you and I love you.
But I am an actor first
You are a lover first
The young man stared into his lover's eyes, and the stewardess called out: Get on the plane.
Come with me. I could not survive the urban jungle. I would turn to stone and you would not love me.
The plane began to leave. The young man was scared but knew what he needed. He threw his things on the plane but decided to stay. He embraced the lover with the black eyes, and they went back where he will teach the children Spanish.
He got letters from home begging him to come back. But he had found his place. He never answered the letters but let them know he was well and happy.
I have found love and I have found life and I will stay.

Michael called this story "*Mi Vida Abajo.*" I asked him to name the roles in the story and speak about them. He named: the beach; the children; the lover, who was pure, loving energy; the questioning, searching young man, who was looking for love and stimulation and nature; the people who write letters; and the stewardess. He specified his sister and parents as the letter writers, and said that he would especially miss his sister. He spoke of the stewardess as his conscience, the part that asks: How could you let go of your actor role?

Far away from the bugs, Michael again created his fantasy world inhabited by innocent characters: a child, a true lover, and a benign, regenerative nature. To have all this, Michael knew that he must give up his attachment to his family, especially his sister, and his professional ambitions to be a great actor. As storyteller, Michael knew that somehow his "life down there" would have to coincide with his "life up here." For the second time he fantasized about teaching children Spanish. What did the child part of himself need to learn? What foreign voice needed to be activated? Perhaps the answers lay in the ambivalences set up by Michael: the innocent child role and the experienced adult role; the romantic, faraway part and the reality of the everyday; healing nature and splitting nurture; the spontaneous one and the actor.

THE CONFUSED SEARCHER

In a subsequent session, the role of the questioning, searching young man became that of the confused searcher, the ambivalent one. The generic searcher role remained as its qualities shifted. I think this happened because Michael was in a new relationship with a man who was a grown-up, genuinely interested in a committed relationship. Although this was potentially vital for Michael, it was also more frightening than ever before.

The new man, Bill, was comfortable in his role as a gay man, involved in organizing political and social events in celebration of being gay. Michael had finally come face to face with a loving, caring, adult father figure. He chose at first to withhold sex, as he often did at the beginning of a new relationship.

I decided to help Michael shift from the fairy-tale, escapist style of "Mi Vida Abajo" and work representationally toward a more direct level of feeling. I asked him to work with three chairs, as we had done in the past. One represented Bill, one stood for Michael, and the third, the chair in the middle, was the narrator, a reflective voice commenting upon the dialogue between Michael and Bill. Michael began as himself:

I wanna be in control. I feel grossed out by sex. I don't know.

(As Bill:) I really like you a lot, but I don't want to get too involved. You're young and I don't know what you want. I feel like I wanna be with you. If you don't wanna have sex, that's OK.

(*As Narrator:*) There's a stand-off. Michael is not dealing with his sexuality. He doesn't know what he's looking for. Bill is a self-contained man. He doesn't want to get hurt. Four days later, they've had sex for the first time. They're lying in bed together.

(*As Michael:*) I don't know what I feel. I feel scared. Hurt. Angry. I don't know where this was coming from. I don't know what to do. (*Michael cried, pointed to his chest.*) I'd like to say I want to be alone, but I don't. I'm afraid. I don't want you to be mad at me. (*He sobbed.*)

(*Michael took on the narrator role, but was unable to speak. He then moved into the role of Bill.*)

(*As Bill:*) I don't want to make you feel any way you don't want to feel. I'm OK with myself and want things to be OK with you.

(*Again, Michael moved to the narrator role, and again fell silent.*)

I asked him to create an image and name for each role. He called the narrator "The Balance," and stretched his arms out wide. He called Bill "The Unsurefooted Appeaser," and reached out in a circular motion with both arms. For the final role, Michael pulled his shirt over his face. He was masked, turned in on himself. His name was "The Confused Searcher."

THE BEAT OF BLACK WINGS

Going deeper into the psyche, Michael reverted back to the presentational quality of myth:

There are many fears in the house. Yet the house was so nice and relaxing. It overlooks the river and trees. You'd think you were in a paradise. You try to make it your web. In the house a Young Man comes to fuck an Older Man. The Young Man felt what it was like to be with someone.

In the house of peace, a scary monster came out of the closet The Older Man had a bad dream. The Young Man pushed them both into the closet and said: Stay in there until you can leave me alone! I just want to stay in peace in this house.

From under the door came black bugs. They circled the Young Man. Help me! Can't you see your fear is getting me? Take them back. I don't want them.

The Older Man said: You have to let me out of the closet first

The Young Man kicked through the circle of bugs and yanked open the closet But only the Older Man was there. The bugs had vanished.

The Older Man said: You see, you have nothing to be afraid of. This house is a safe house.

I don't trust you any more, said the Young Man. You brought on these monsters.

But the Young Man couldn't leave because there was a storm outside. He didn't want to be touched by the Older Man.

In the morning it was tranquil. Was this all a nightmare? There were only clothes in the closet. The bed was made, and it seemed that no one had laid in it. The Young Man got dressed, opened the window, and saw a slight piece of wing from a black bug. He threw the wing out the window and watched it turn over and over, catching the sunlight, fluttering until it reached the ground. He felt something in his heart. Was it fear? As the wing caught the sun, it turned gold. It wasn't fear alone. Just as the Young Man knew what it was, the sun blinded him and made him forget. So the Young Man waited for the Older Man to come back, but he didn't come. He waited and waited and wondered if it really happened at all.

Michael told this story, which he called "The Beat of Black Wings," after actually spending a night with Bill. They had had satisfying sex with Michael taking on both passive and active roles. Long after falling asleep, Bill woke up in a panic, screaming. Michael became very frightened. He got up out of bed and went to the bathroom down the hall, fearful that he would encounter a water bug. When he turned on the bathroom light, a large water bug appeared. Michael became terrified, turned off the light, and ran back toward the bedroom without daring to kill the bug. While in his panic, he became aware that someone had turned on the bathroom light. He turned around and saw Bill, who somehow had gotten out of bed and into the bathroom. Michael just wanted to sleep it off. He did not ask Bill about his nightmare. They both eventually fell asleep, without talking about the incident.

Michael identified the following roles in the story: the Young Man, the Older Man, the scary monster, the black bugs, and the wing. He did not initially mention the house, the sun, or the closet.

He called the Young Man a confused searcher, whose purpose was to search for a safe home, a loving place. He is open and trusting but confused. En-roled as the Young Man, Michael said:

I don't know what I feel. I feel scared. Hurt. Angry. I don't know where this was coming from.

The Older Man is also a searcher, but he is more complex. On the one hand, according to Michael, he is "searching for the end of the rainbow," but on the other hand, he is the keeper of the scary monster. There is an undercurrent to him; something is not completely safe. Without the Older Man, there would be no scary monster.

Michael left the scary monster somewhat undefined. All he said was that the monster knows when to come to the Young Man and that the Young Man can call him up at any time. In my own mind, I related the scary monster back to the Black Rage, the terrifying power of his father. The screams of Bill might provoke a reaction in Michael similar to that of the Black Rage; if this was the case, such terrors would need to be shut up in the closet.

As Michael saw it, the little bit of wing is something left behind by the scary monster. It has a supernatural power and is part of the terror. Yet it is also transformed by the sun into something beautiful, which, to Michael, is "like a gift or angel trying to show something."

Michael also addressed the roles not initially mentioned:

> The sun is the healer. It can shine light or make love in places of darkness. It can establish trust and impart knowledge where once there was confusion.

The closet is the lair of the scary monster, the domain of fear.

I asked Michael which character he felt closest to. He answered:

> The sun . . . the safety and the distance that I have now. There's always a bit of black wing.

How does the sun serve you in your life?

> I am like the sun, the part that will protect me. Maybe there's too much protection. Maybe that's the black wing . . . pulling back and opening up, fear versus life.

Going further, Michael wondered whether he needed more than protection:

> I want to blame the other one for making me sad and angry and mistrustful, but I don't know. I'm angry that I'm not saved by the sun or the Older Man. It's gonna be work. I wanna be taken care of. (*He was lying on the floor and had assumed the fetal position.*) I feel that the black bug was sexual. Sexual terror . . .

I asked him to take on the role of a black bug, the one role he had neglected to reflect upon:

> I don't know. I am the black bug. I come out of the darkness. I move very slowly. I'm only looking to fulfill my needs. I come out of the darkness. Looking for . . . looking for . . . I don't know what I'm looking for. When you're unprotected, I walk across your arm, across your mouth in your sleep. If you admit that you want it, you might not be afraid. I creep. I'm looking to fulfill my needs. If I touch you, you will not die. I can be beautiful if you look

at me. Then you try to kill me and I'm very afraid. I must die because of your fear. To die because of fear—that is my legacy.

The legacy of the black bug is the legacy of the Black Rage, one of a paralyzing fear that can kill all chance of sexual and filial love. With the role of the bug, however, Michael provided the possibility of transformation through the image of the sunlight on the wing. "I can be beautiful if you look at me," he said. If he could indeed see fully and admit the powerful role of fear into his life, then the legacy of Black Rage could be transformed. When I asked Michael what he would call the transformation, he responded: "A life of love." That life remained elusive, but was suddenly possible. Bill was not his father, and Michael recognized this. He knew, too, that he had the power to defeat bugs, or at the very least to confront them.

MY FATHER'S BODY

Bill was a lawyer, 45 years old. The lawyer's function as defender and protector of victims falsely accused was strongly embedded in Michael's mind. However, the fact that Bill, like his father, was attractive, hairy, masculine, and older weighed heavily upon Michael. Even though he was now aware, in part, of how his father intruded upon his intimate and sexual life, the struggle for effective, nonincestuous relationships was just beginning. Bill was carrying the projections not only of Michael's father, but also of Julian and all the fantasy lawyers who might be available to rescue the innocent victim, Michael, from his own emotional and moral demons.

Sex was wonderful with Bill, when it was the right time of day in the right bed (Bill's), when the sheets were clean, and when their bodies were freshly showered. For Michael, there were many prohibitions and ambivalences, the most nagging of which concerned who was on top and who was on bottom. Michael generally took on the submissive sexual role, but in his sexual relationship with Bill, he was given permission to take on the dominant role. Although it was erotic and powerful, Michael experienced a certain repulsion. In dominant sex, Michael became so identified with his father that he feared the loss of his feminine, innocent side. On the other hand, when he assumed the passive role, he became like his mother, whom he imagined to be passive in bed, letting go of the control she exerted in so many other aspects of her life. The passive role was frightening because it provoked incestuous fears.

Michael was in a sexual dilemma. Neither of his two sexual role models appeared to be appropriate. The father's sexual power was that of the aggressive, violent castrator. In Michael's mind, the mother, who also had the power to castrate, had already emasculated the father. Her methods were: criticizing him to death and taking away his power and self-respect; she left him, in effect, with a small masculine triumph—the right to be on top when in bed. Reiterating his sexual fears and lack of sexual expertise, Michael said: "Instead of sex, I had sterility."

In a dream, Michael was outside of his house and there were many holes in the lawn. His father warned him to be careful of the holes. When I asked him to speak from the point of view of the holes, Michael charged them with a direct sexuality. The holes in the ground were the domains of the sexual demons that plagued Michael. In the earlier story, the scary monster with its attendant bugs also belongs to the province of the father. The attraction and repulsion of the father's body dominated Michael's sexual relationship with Bill.

I asked Michael to speak of his father's body, in a kind of litany:

My father's body is hairy. My father's body is scary. My father's body is gross. My father's body is tight. My father's body is fleshy. My father's body is smelly. My father's body is hard. My father's body is sweaty. My father's body is annoying. My father's body is always naked. My father's body is hairy and scary. My father's body is sexual. My father's body is attractive. My father's body is always naked. My father's body is always parading around. My father's body is in the way when I'm watching television. My father's body wants me to look at it. My father's body is selfish. My father's body is young. My father's body is annoying. My father's body is hairy. My father's body is scary.

Yet again Michael was a young boy in bed with his mother, both attracted and repelled by his father's exhibitionism. The attraction was toward the male, sexual, almost godlike presence of the father. The repulsion was toward the unnatural demands that his father's sexual presence made upon him: to look and perhaps even to satisfy both father's and son's incestuous wishes.

Michael then told this story:

Once upon a time there was a little boy and he had a father who always paraded around like a peacock, showing off his feathers. The neighbors always said to him: What a nice body you have!

One day the boy said to his father: You have a nice body.

The father responded: You're not supposed to say that.

The boy thought he was strange because he noticed what a beautiful body his father had. Each time he complemented his father, he was scold-

ed, so he said: You have an ugly body, gross and disgusting, and I hate it and I hate you!

The father replied: You don't know anything about bodies. I have a beautiful body. Go to your room!

While in his room, the boy thought: I hate your body. It's ugly and scary.

One day the boy grew into a young man. The father's body had aged. The young man thought he had the wrong kind of body. One hot day he walked into the house with few clothes on and his father said: You have a beautiful body.

The young man replied: You're not supposed to notice a boy's body.

The boy looked into the mirror and wanted to knew if his body was beautiful or ugly. The people outside thought it was beautiful.

One day, the boy met a man with a body like his father. The man liked his body and he liked the man's body. They put their bodies together and enjoyed each other.

Sometimes it came into his head that the man's body was ugly because it was like his father's body.

Michael entitled the story "The Emperor's New Body." The title seems ironic because in the original, "The Emperor's New Clothes," the innocent young boy was able to see through the hypocrisy and foolishness of the adults. In Michael's story, the boy and the adult figures of father and townspeople (chorus) are confusing and they pass on their confusion to the boy. In fact, in the story as Michael told it, the boy and the young man that he becomes are confused. The vision of the boy/young man and the vision of the father/chorus are the same.

The one adult role offering help to the confused boy is that of the man with a body like his father's. But the helper role is ineffective, as it is too closely linked in the boy's mind with the body of the father.

Again we see Michael's profound ambiguities brought about by a father who both taught the incest taboo and then violated his own teaching. The ambiguities of father and lover, good body and bad body, the beautiful and the repulsive, the boy and the man abound in this story.

After sex with Bill, as had been the case after sex with other men, Michael felt an immediate compulsion to shower and change the sheets. If he was to spend the night with Bill, he steeled himself against the prospect that Bill would demand sexual favors in the morning. Michael remained too exposed to the father role, which in this case was too inconsistent, overpowering, and threatening. The image of the father that Michael had internalized did not serve him well at all. It functioned to sabotage each potentially intimate sexual relationship he had with another man. It functioned to keep him mired in the fears of castration and in sexual, moral, and emotional ambivalence. In order to proceed toward a functional intimate and sexual relationship with another man, Michael needed to move beyond the small transformation of the little bit of wing; the father role that lived inside Michael needed to be reconceived and transformed.

MICKEY AND JAKE:
YOU DREAM AT YOUR OWN RISK

Michael was slipping. His external life had become busy, with too many temp jobs and a role in a small play about Vietnam. He canceled a number of therapy appointments and expressed much ambivalence about Bill. While visiting his family during the Thanksgiving holidays, he found himself in the house one night, alone and lonely; instead of calling Bill, he phoned the older man on the sex line, who offered a very safe and temporarily satisfying sexual encounter.

Michael was displeased with his role in the play. He had auditioned for both roles: Jake, a prototypical hurt child, fearful and suspicious, trapped in a minefield in Vietnam with no inner resources; and Mickey, a protector and caretaker, a powerful, heroic type, who has inner resources that he uses in his quest to return home. There is a third offstage character in the play, Rogers, a displaced person who cannot survive the chaos of war, yet is equally unfit to survive the bourgeois placidity of home. Although the character never appears, Michael also identified with Rogers.

His audition was good enough to land him the role of Jake, which he coveted. But the director gave a weaker actor the Jake role. Michael was cast as Mickey. He resented the director for her casting mistake. Like his mother, she did not give him what he wanted; that was, she did not reward his behavior as an angry, hurt child. He also resented the actor playing Jake for his professional incompetence and awkwardness, as well as for exhibiting overtly gay mannerisms. Even the stage manager became an object of Michael's wrath. He was an older man who one day stood in for the actor playing Jake and overzealously pushed Michael hard against a wall, following a stage direction in the script to the letter. Like his father, the stage manager physically abused Michael, unwittingly, in a role he had no business assuming. When Michael confronted him, the stage manager answered:

> But I'm not an actor. How can you expect me to know how hard to push you? I was just following the script.

For Michael that response echoed his father's (see Chapter Four):

> But I was just a child myself. . . . You can't expect me to be differ-
> ent [i.e., behave like a father].

Most of all, Michael resented not being allowed to play the role of the hurt child—the one most closely linked to his own resentment toward those who had figuratively forced him into an emotional minefield, abandoning him there with no effective defense.

In preparing emotionally for the role of Mickey, Michael imagined that his brother was trapped in the minefield and he must save him. While at home for Thanksgiving, he even asked Steve to scream on a tape recorder to provide a more heightened sense of emotional reality. He further imagined that his sister Bea, like Rogers, got killed foolishly and that he was angry at her and at himself for being unable to save her. For Michael, the boundaries between fiction and everyday reality were narrow.

I asked Michael to improvise a dialogue between the characters of Jake and Mickey:

> JAKE: I am alive. I don't wanna face my fear. I don't wanna die. I just wanna get out of here and lie down.
>
> MICKEY: They hurt me. I'm hurt and I'm tired of being hurt. I'm gonna walk into the fire. Hit me, Daddy, I don't care. Fuckin' hit me! I'm not gonna change. I'm not gonna be hurt. I'm gonna get my baby out of here. There's a part of me that still can feel and still can hurt. I'm gonna get that part away from you. I don't care if I die. I don't care any more, Daddy. Fuckin' shoot me! I can die.
>
> JAKE: I don't wanna die. I'm tired. I just wanna lie down. I'm afraid. I don't wanna know any more.
>
> MICKEY: Come on, get the fuck up, you fuckin' lazy pig. Get up. I'm gonna yank you by the hair. Get the fuck up! Get up! Please, please. Don't give up. Please, I'm begging. I'm not going on without you. You fuckin' lazy pig. I wanna give up, too, you know. But I can't. I'm not gonna give them the satisfaction. I'm not lying down for anybody. You fuckin' call me a fag, Daddy, I'm not lying down for you. Get up, please! . . . If I lie down for one minute, will you get up?
>
> JAKE: What if I can't get up again? I'm afraid. Get me home. Just get me home!
>
> MICKEY: I can't lie down any more. I don't know how. I'm gonna try. I'm gonna try to lie down.
>
> JAKE: If I can't get up again? . . . (*Michael cried.*) Help me!

In the dialogue, Mickey is ambivalent. On the one hand, he is a warrior and survivor, determined to overcome the abuses of his father, save his partner, and conquer death. When he says, "I'm gonna get my baby out of here," he refers to the feeling part of himself, which refuses to shut down in the face of violence and threat. On the other hand, he is worn out, shut down, fearful that he can't make it alone.

By contrast, the Jake role becomes minor. Michael had moved beyond the whimpering, needy child. He was cast in the role of Mickey for a good reason: He was ready. The adult role was an ambivalent one and a real stretch. It was a rehearsal for a life as an adult. Michael recognized that the Mickey part of himself was stronger than the Jake part. A shift had occurred.

Michael characterized Mickey as tired of being afraid; he actually strived to get home. The play was about to open, and he was beginning to feel secure in the role. One line continued to baffle him, however. It refers to Rogers, who is discharged from the army but returns to the battlefield after failing to make it in the domestic world back home. Back on the front lines, he meets a violent death. The baffling line is "You dream at your own risk."

For the first time in our work together, Michael spoke about God and death. He mentioned that he felt closer to allowing himself to be tested for AIDS. He seemed willing to risk more than ever before. I asked Michael to create a story about Mickey and Rogers, incorporating the confusing line: "You dream at your own risk."

There was this soldier, Mickey, fighting in Vietnam. He didn't know why or who he was fighting, but he knew he had to get home. He was afraid of the jungles and the sounds. He heard this voice and it said: Don't be afraid any more. All you need to know is me.

He turned around. There were two energies, one bright and glowing, which said: No matter what you do, you'll end up here with me. I'm what you call God.

The other was dark and said: Go forward and I'll follow you. Just take a step.

Mickey ran. He was confused and ran until he found Rogers, who said: I just saw a bright light which said not to be afraid any more, that I would be all right. I tried to follow it but it kept moving. I was standing in this dark cloud, but I couldn't get out . . . I don't wanna die.

Mickey said: Don't be afraid any more.

Rogers said: I'm so afraid, I don't know where I'm going.

Mickey asked: What are you afraid of?

Rogers said: I don't know. I thought I had it all—wife, money, love, fame, but I went back there and it just stared at me and I stared at it, but it didn't touch me any more. I needed to drive in a fast car. I just needed to be scared.

Mickey asked: What does that mean?
Rogers said: I don't know.
Mickey said: You're crazy. Why do you want to be afraid?
Rogers said: Because when you're afraid you know the truth. Fear is the truth.
Mickey said: Fear is not the truth.
Rogers held up a gun. He said: I have this gun with one bullet I'm gonna spin the cartridge and shoot once.
Mickey said: You're crazy.
Rogers spun the cartridge. He pulled the trigger. It clicked and he laughed.
Mickey said: You fuckin' asshole.
Rogers said: Nothing touches me any more.
Mickey ran and ran and was afraid someone was going to jump out and shoot him. He heard a bang and a cry and knew Rogers had killed himself. He stared at the woods and saw the black clouds above. He said: I'm not afraid of you. I'm not gonna let you take me.
He ran through smoke and bugs and rats eating out dismembered body parts, until he saw the light As he was about to reach it, the light vanished. All was quiet A voice came back and said: What do you need?
Mickey held out his outstretched palm and said: You tell me what I need.
The voice said: You have to know.
Mickey sat there with his hands held up to the sky. He was numb inside. The thunder and lightning came closer and closer. One raindrop fell into his palm; it ran down his wrist and he asked: Why did you give me a raindrop?
The voice said: Because this is all you are.
He thought he understood that there was no answer. He laughed and the sky rumbled. He cried and the rain fell on him. He laughed and cried; it rained and thundered. The sun came out and he grew peaceful inside. He opened his eyes and saw Rogers, standing in front of him. He said: Hey, Rogers, I think I understand.
Rogers stood there with a hole in his head. He said: Don't you see? You shouldn't have wanted it to touch you. You should have touched it first When you actually do it, you make it When you dream of it touching you, you do so at your own risk.

Michael saw Rogers's message, delivered from beyond the grave, as concerning the risks of the passive life. The dreamer part of Michael functioned to kept him within a passive mode. Indulging in fantasies of the perfect home, the perfect father and lover, kept Michael in his emotional minefield. When he dreamed this kind of dream, he risked losing the active, adult part of himself, represented by Mickey—the part that would continue to search for ways out of all fearful battlefields.

In the context of the characters in the play, the risk for Michael was that of never getting home. Within the story, he presented several parts of himself. One, again represented by Mickey, is the hero on a spiritual search. This role functions to move him to a truth beyond fear, through the minefields and horrifying landscapes, toward the light of reason and hope.

Another, represented by Rogers, is the coward, one who has given up hope, accepting the dictum that truth is fear. Having pursued his material dreams and judged them empty, he returns to the battlefield, the only place available for him to feel fully alive. His risky dancing on the edge of the grave proves deadly. He becomes a suicide, later resurrected to bring back a moral from the grave: You dream at your own risk.

The Rogers part of Michael was what kept him in his fear and despair. Living the fearful life was comfortable for Michael, as was the image of himself as the wounded, emotionally dead victim. The Rogers part of Michael also reminded him of his ambivalent quest for recognition and ideal love. It fueled the despair that he generally felt by reminding him that even if he were to make it, the emptiness inside would still compel him to commit self-destructive acts.

Rogers's posthumous message, however, reveals another side of Michael and provides some real sustenance. In a way, he urges Michael to reject passivity and do battle with the forces of darkness. His message echoes the lines of Dylan Thomas (1957, p. 128):

> Do not go gentle into that good night . . .
> Rage, rage against the dying of the light.

As in the earlier story, "The Beat of Black Wings," there are natural and supernatural roles at work. The forces of light are the healers. In "The Beat of Black Wings," the wing of a black bug is transformed into a thing of beauty by the sun. Here, too, the sun brings tranquility and peace. And in the presence of God, Mickey is compared to a raindrop, a perfect piece of nature. Mickey is liberated, allowing his emotions to flow freely, like the rain and the thunder.

The natural and supernatural roles offer a transcendence of fear through love. And thus we come to the end of the story of Rogers, who urges Mickey to be the one to touch it, in reality. In Michael's life, "it" represents the things that he was most afraid of: the bugs, AIDS, the Black Rage, the body of the father, the hand of God that might mask the face of Death. In the previous story, Michael as a black bug had said: "If I touch you, you will not die." Here again, he conveyed that message: Touch does not kill; in fact, it is natural and healing. The transcendent parts of Michael were available to deliver this message to the part of Michael that was awake. The challenge was for the speaking part and the listening part to communicate. In hearing, Michael discovered the meaning of the line: You dream at your own risk. He was a little bit more awake now and less at risk of losing his bearings in his self-constructed minefield.

VICTIM/VICTIMIZER/VICTOR

Again the dreamworld appeared, signaled by Rogers's line: "Nothing touches me any more." Michael retreated to the role of the outsider, the voyeur, secure in his isolation, shielded by his judgment of others. He told me of his disappointments with Bill, whom he saw as weak, unsuccessful, and unambitious as a lawyer, too much the victim, not enough the defender he should be. Michael so very much needed others to be consistent with their roles: A lawyer should be strong and protective, as should a father.

Back to phone sex, Michael removed himself even further from the older man on the line by listening to recorded messages of men advertising themselves—perfect sexual objects, twice removed. He dreamed at his own risk.

He had a dream about Bea. She met Michael in a Chinese restaurant (where he was, in fact, to meet Bill) and verbally abused him, humiliating him terribly. Her voice hit Michael with all the power of the Black Rage.

Then something shifted. There was no great catharsis, no explosive realization. The small increments of his therapeutic work during the past 2 years simply added up. He decided to leave the city for a time and journey to Spain where he would study Spanish. The play ended and the role of Mickey felt more solidly integrated for him—Mickey as adult, as survivor, and man of action.

Michael spoke to Bill about his feelings for the first time. It was the holiday season and they were about to go to the country for the weekend with a group of Bill's friends, all gay men. Michael was afraid that he would lose control and be seduced—that is, victimized or at least estranged, lost in the meeting of men. He told Bill that he was scared, that he feared losing control so far away from home. Bill said little, but held Michael and reassured him that he cared about him and would never hurt him. Michael accepted this message.

One night, Michael and Bill were in bed. There was a snowstorm. Bill wanted to make love, but Michael was ambivalent. He moved away, complaining of a neckache. Bill massaged him gently and Michael cried. Then they were both silent. Michael moved away and watched the city fill up with snow. Nature again covered, touched, healed.

In therapy, Michael presented his dilemma as clearly as ever:

When I become engaged sexually, I need to disengage emotionally. Because when I allow myself to be intimate, I feel victimized.

Michael said that he was at the heart of his issue with his father. In attempting intimacy with his father, he received abuse. The intimacy was tied into incestuous fantasies. Thus, sex and violence became paired, as did intimacy and self-protective distance.

For Michael, this knowledge was beginning to lead to an understanding and revision of his roles of victim, intimate, and sexual lover. In spite of all his retreats into overdistanced roles, he was sustaining a relationship with a "good enough" (see Winnicott, 1971) man, and was discovering the potential of the adult part of himself that could father, protect, and sustain him throughout many dark and stormy nights.

He went further. Now that the demonic power of the father was clearer, he raged against the power of the mother. He saw her now as even more powerful than the father who easily played victim to her victimizer role. Her power lay in words that withered his physical threats: "If you touch me, I will leave you for good."

Touch, then, could kill, or at least threaten a relationship. In taking on both the part of the father who touched abusively and the mother who overcame the fear of abusive touch through threats of abandonment, Michael had developed his own ambivalences in regard to intimacy.

Michael's sense of power and control had in large measure been taken on from his mother. On the one hand, she was the ultimate critic, absolute in her thinking. If men were too threatening, either through violence or sex, she abandoned them. In his relationship with Bill, Michael exercised this warning: "Touch me the wrong way and I'm gone."

Furthermore, the mother was unmatched in her use of words as weapons. Like his role model, Michael took on the role of witty fool to practice the ways he thought women control men. As fool, he assumed a lowly status and wielded a sharp tongue in order to control those whom he deemed more powerful than he. His method, like Hamlet's, was indirect, antic, and cutting. The two victimizer roles—that of the physically abusive, direct father and that of the verbally abusive, indirect mother—held Michael in his victim role, shielding him from intimacy.

Shortly before leaving for his trip to the country with the group of men, he had a dream:

A woman friend of mine is up on a ledge, a platform near the ceiling of my room in the city. I am below, watching, though fearful that she is too close to the places where the roaches and other bugs nest. The woman had given birth to a baby, which appeared to be a false baby. She handed it down to me. Another woman, an actress, is trying to get in touch with her feelings in an acting class. Her teacher is nearby, though a vague presence. Bugs appear near the woman on the ledge. They are everywhere. I crush them all. Then I say: I've got to move.

Among the characters in this dream story, Michael felt closest to the role of himself, which he characterized as that of the voyeur— that is, until the voyeur assumes the warrior role and exterminates the bugs. He felt most distant from the role of the teacher, whom he characterized as the alleged enlightened one. In a dialogue between the two characters, the following emerged:

VOYEUR: Teacher, why are you standing back so far? Why don't you do something? Why are you letting the actress just stand there all alone with her feelings?

TEACHER: What do you want from me? Everyone wants me to show them the way. I can give you a few pushes here and there. But she's got to find her way on her own. Why are you worried about her? She's up there trying. You're the one who's standing back and watching. You've got to kill some bugs. Do something. Stop worrying about her and her distanced feelings.

VOYEUR: I'm tired of these fucking bugs. They're in the way. I can't get through the door. You're no help. I've gotta kill these bugs. They're not in my room at home. Actress, get down from there. Aren't you afraid of the bugs? What if the baby gets killed by the bugs?

I asked Michael to take on other roles, as he chose.

BABY: That guy's freaking out. He's so crazy. Everything's fine for me. I'm not afraid.

BUG: Moisture, moisture. Warmth. (*Michael crawled on the floor.*) Little baby's not afraid of bugs. Baby's not afraid of bugs . . .

Michael de-roled and spoke of the connection between the dream roles and himself. He specified the bugs as both victimizers and victims. The bugs suddenly appear and frighten people. Yet in the face of children (in this case, the baby), their power is diminished. As victimizers, spreaders of fear, they also embody the qualities of victims, vulnerable themselves to innocence and to fear (as Michael noted earlier in taking the role of a black bug: "Then you try to kill me and I'm very afraid"). Furthermore, as the warrior part of Michael becomes activated in the dream, the bugs are crushed. Perhaps the dreaded bugs were steadily losing their power over Michael.

When I first met Michael, he was carrying around the story of "Beauty and the Beast." More and more, the bug role resembled that of the Beast, a pariah of great power, one capable of victimizing others. Yet, below the surface, this fairy-tale Beast is himself a victim, an abused prince cast in a evil spell, capable of loving if only an inno-cent beauty can save him from his false role through her loyalty and love. In the dream, the bug/beast finds its neutralizer, the baby.

The baby was the innocent, according to Michael. He sees no evil, not even in the bugs; yet he needs protection. Again, this innocent role was one Michael had been working through for some time, most clearly in his extensive cast of child characters. The baby part of Michael functioned to keep him in his dreams of perfection. When enacted alone, the role was too passive and vulnerable. In the dream, the protection comes in the form of the bug/beast, which allows the innocent to survive. Within the fearful symmetry of innocent–beast, Michael could discover a means of living in the ambivalence of open-ness and fear.

The baby in Michael's dream is seen as potentially false, signify-ing the potentially false innocence that subsisted within Michael. Michael was slowly becoming aware that when he played out the in-nocent role, he was expressing not only the romantic qualities of fairy-tale figures, but also a manipulative quality that served to get him what he wanted.

According to Michael, the teacher is the adult, capable of assert-ing his needs. He possesses some wisdom, being allegedly en-lightened, but also is quick to turn people in the direction of their own wisdom. This role is dimly envisioned in the dream because Michael often doubted the existence of the adult part of himself. Yet, in his struggle to be the adult, he was learning to assert his needs to Bill.

Michael described the actress role as the part of himself strug-gling to express feelings. Like the innocent, it is vulnerable and in need of another for sustenance. The image of the mother giving birth to the baby mirrors the actress role giving birth to her feelings. The teacher, a version of the adult/father role, is present to help baby the feelings along. The part of Michael that was the actress struggled con-stantly with the birthing of feelings. In many ways, he had chosen this role professionally as a way of procreating. The femininity of the dream actress is significant in reinforcing Michael's need to express his feminine side, full of feeling and nurturance.

Michael viewed the function of the mother role, the woman on the ledge, as giving birth and handing the baby down to Michael. She is the source of innocence and creativity, virtues to be passed on to Michael. She remains close to the bugs/fears as she performs her function, but reproduces life nonetheless. Although Michael recognized this part of himself as sometimes remote and fearful, he also acknowledged his need to get closer to his own source of creativity.

The final role of Michael as voyeur is a very familiar one. In the dream, the voyeur stands back and accuses others (e.g., the teacher) of not solving the bug problem for him. He complains and whines and longs for the safe house of his childhood. Yet, unlike the over-distanced quality that appears in many other dramas, this angry, hurt child/victim rises to the occasion, heroically kills the bugs, and is ready to move on. The victim has become victor. And, according to Michael, the victor is a survivor, one who has successfully waged a moral battle and is ready to move on.

In working through this dream, Michael established the connections between beauty and beast; student and teacher; baby and mother; and victim, victimizer, and victor. Michael held the child, passed down from the ledge, in his hands, as he had once before cradled Patty, the mute, victimized part of himself. As this child (which Michael called "the baby of disbelief"), he spoke, saying that he was not afraid. In acting, killing the bugs, he transformed the several passive roles of voyeur, dreamer, and victim. Michael discovered that on the other side of these passive roles lay those not only of victor and survivor, but also of hero, one who engages in risky but brave journeys toward self-discovery. Because his role system had changed, his heroic journey into the ambiguities of intimacy was to assume new dimensions.

THE RING

The ring was the initial image that arose in our work together. It was chosen as a role by Michael from "Beauty and the Beast." It remained a mystery to me for some 2 years in terms of type, quality, and function. At the beginning of Chapter Four, I have spoken of the ring as a bond between father and daughter, as a bond between Beauty and Beast, and as a transitional object that allows Beauty to break with the father and move toward the lover.

In moving toward the final stages of therapy, Michael spoke of the ring again. He called it a talisman, a unifier, a complete circle encompassing all of his roles. A story followed:

Once upon a time, there was a shiny golden ring, forged in a mixture of hot, burning fire and cold ice. The marriage of fire and ice yields a middle ground of pure gold. The ring was sold to a king who had every material thing one could think of. When he put on the ring, he had great wisdom. When his subjects came to him with difficult questions, he put on the ring and always gave perfect answers. It was festival time and there was a big parade. Accidentally, the ring flew off the king's finger, without his knowledge. When the people around him asked questions, he answered in a confused way. He finally became aware of the loss of the ring and desperately searched everywhere. But the ring had rolled beyond the parade, to the feet of a young man weeping on a street corner. He picked up the ring and it shone as bright as the sun in his eyes. The ring asked the young man: Why are you crying?

He responded: Because the parade passed me by.

The young man put the ring on his thumb and walked home. He felt powerful and wise. People began to notice him and followed after. Groups began to form and whisper among themselves: Who is this young man? The king appeared and was also impressed by this very special young man. The people raised him on their shoulders and honored him.

I'm not watching the parade; I am the parade, he said.

Suddenly, the ring flew off his finger onto the ground. The people stared and recognized it as the king's ring. They dropped the young man and called him thief. They dragged him before the king, who said: You stole my ring. For this you shall be punished by death.

The king picked up his ring, then looked up at the boy being taken to his death. He called out: Wait! Bring him back. And to the boy he said: Where did you get this ring?

The boy said: It came to me suddenly, and I understood what it was like to get what I needed.

The king replied: I will let you live, but on one condition: You must become a prince and live all your years as my son.

The young man sobbed and realized he wouldn't miss his past life as a depressed, self-pitying person. A crown was brought in, and the young man became prince of the kingdom. The king called a welder and asked him to divide the ring into two thin bands of bright light and gold. And so the king and prince each wore a part of the ring and lived happily ever after.

As Michael now saw it, the ring is the creative principle that holds contradictions and transforms passivity into action, ignorance into wisdom, death into love, isolation into connection.

At this point in time, the wheel had come full circle regarding Michael's relationship to his father. Earlier, we have seen Michael's grave sexual fear of a castrating father who forced his son into the role of victim. We have seen Michael's attempts to confront his father, only to meet with the realization that the father had no idea how to assume the adult role. And we have seen his thwarted attempts to realize his adult sexuality in the face of men who, like his father, would prove ultimately repulsive and unacceptable. The only father figure whom Michael could safely embrace was an anonymous older man who talked erotically on a telephone sex line.

With the slow acceptance of Bill, the wheel moved closer to connecting Michael with the acceptable qualities of the father. Bill as symbolic father was protective, slow and steady, gentle and nurturing. Furthermore, he was politically connected to a larger group of peers, a kind of "generalized other" who might serve Michael as a positive role model. In journeying to the country during the New Year's holidays, fearful of being abused by the potentially Dionysian group and being thrust yet again into the helpless victim role, Michael was delighted to discover a camaraderie and to be ritually inducted into a group of peers. He found himself in a ritual sweathouse, sitting naked with the other men around a steamy fire and feeling a sense of contentment and belonging. He was with others who were like him in essential ways. If they touched him, he did not have to be afraid. Their touch would be neither lethal nor rageful. He had his lawyer with him, and his many childlike roles; he even had his own ability, perhaps for the first time, to father himself.

In the story of the ring, the king/father and the lonely boy/son are united. On one level, the ring of father and son indicates that Michael had resolved his essential conflict with his father. The king/father, not having recognized the lonely boy/son as his own and having abused him through condemning him to death, renounces his mistaken vision. The ring of wisdom allows him to see the truth and save both the son and the relationship. Father and son are reconciled and will share the power, the home, the wisdom.

On another level, the ring shows that an inner circle was completed. The part of Michael that was brutal, confusing, and incestuous had loosened its hold over the part that was isolated, estranged, and totally vulnerable. The victimizing part of Michael had made peace with the victim part. Michael now had a new way to protect and nurture himself, mirroring Bill's positive fathering and the ongoing fathering offered through the therapeutic process.

I asked Michael to make a drawing of the significant people in his life. He placed himself at the center. Bill was the closest of all and loomed large. His mother was the farthest away, but his father was not even on the page. The actual father no longer controlled Michael with an abusive power. The virtual father inside was equally pushed back to the sidelines.

Michael had learned to be sexual with Bill, unashamed to make love to an older man. The ambivalence remained as he sought out an occasional anonymous yet safe sexual encounter, but he remained fully in the relationship with Bill, learning to accept the mix of revulsion and nurturance. When things got too close, he wavered on the edge of the Black Rage, then caught himself before he fell. And to his dismay and delight, Bill allowed it to happen. Even when with Bill, he still fantasized about being in bed alone again, safe and secure in his pristine sheets. To be *and* not to be at the same time, that was the answer.

Michael was about to embark on the journey prophesied in *"Mi Vida Abajo."* He would study Spanish and try to build a new profession for himself as a bilingual teacher, one who could communicate in two languages. He would allow Bill to visit but would remain distant from his family. His interest in the perfect lover with the black eyes had waned. When he returned, he wanted to work further in therapy on his relationship with his mother—a source of his judgment, resentment, and guilt.

The one language he had known all his life was inherited from his family—that born in fear and rage, spoken by tyrant and victim. The new language, very much in process, was that which could be spoken by a hero, one who would take his ambivalence with him, secure in the knowledge that this was the baggage required for such journeys. At this point of embarkation, a transformed role system had emerged.

POSTSCRIPT

Upon the return from his 4-month journey, Michael felt clearer than ever before. He maintained his relationship with Bill to the extent that he was able to tell him tearfully, "I love you." This was the first time Michael had said that to anybody. In his dreams and conscious confrontations with bugs, Michael survived well. They were still frightening, but Michael had the power to resist and strike back. Of more profound significance, Michael finally took the dreaded AIDS test, willing as never before to face his mortality. With this step, Michael acknowledged perhaps the most feared primary role—that of the mortal, one whose body would ultimately break down. He also recognized that he had held on to the sick, hypochondriacal role because it allowed him to receive nurturance from his mother and saved him from having to grow up and make healthy, adult choices. Upon learning that he tested negative, Michael cried for a long time; embraced Bill, who was there waiting; and went off with his lover to celebrate.

On a professional level, Michael was ready to take a step beyond what he now characterized as the narcissistic profession of acting. He wanted to use the new languages he had learned—that of Spanish, and that of the responsible adult. He intended to enroll in law school and defend those in need. He was ready to continue his hero's journey, hopeful that at the end of this next voyage, he would become a model for others.

The drama therapy role method was effectively employed with Michael as he worked through a variety of roles and came to understand their functions within his life. The often complex intermingling of roles during this process points to the difficulties in applying the method in a direct, linear fashion. However, the process was effective in that it helped Michael move beyond the position of victim, one controlled by overpowering forces (fathers, mothers, and symbolic parents). Yet before arriving at the heroic place of survivor or victor, Michael needed to work through the ways that he victimized himself by holding onto passive, fearful, and depressive roles within. His helpers, in the guise of lawyers, protective judges, lovers, and peers, could only assist him when he was willing to confront the internal demonic forces.

It is not only the transformation from a distressful role to a fulfilling one that marks the effectiveness of the drama therapy process. Its effectiveness will ultimately be measured over time by one's ability to live in the ambivalence of such conflicting roles as victim and victor—a struggle that, although brought to consciousness and marked by a change of behavior, needs to be revisited from time to time like a familiar tale that never quite loses its appeal. For if one treats a transformed role system like a closed book, it may revert back to its previous hold on one's well-being.

In the case example provided in the next chapter, a familiar tale served as a way of looking at another person's journey from victim to survivor. This time, the therapeutic story was told within the context of a group.

CHAPTER SIX

The Case of Hansel and Gretel: An Example of a Drama Therapy Group

This chapter illustrates the dramatic role method as applied to a group drama therapy process. This particular group of eight adults, several of whom had grown up in dysfunctional families, had been together for 1 year. At this point in their process, the group members were working with archetypal stories that encapsulated their own personal concerns. The central figure in the work described here was Ann, a 30-year-old adult child of an alcoholic father. Ann chose the story of "Hansel and Gretel" for the group to dramatize.

The fact that the group used a known story offers another approach to working with role types. As described in Chapters Four and Five, Michael improvised most of his stories, spontaneously invoking the needed role types. This time, the role types exemplified by Hansel and Gretel, among other characters in the story, are based in a fictional narrative that is commonplace within a culture. The roles invoked by group members came conceivably from two places: externally, from the known story, and internally, as identifications were made with the fictional characters in the story.

I again use a storytelling and interpretive approach to reveal the therapeutic role process experienced by Ann and her peers. Ann told her stories on two levels: that of her version of Hansel and Gretel, and that of her actual past experience, told in third person as if it were a fairy tale. The latter was provoked in the telling and dramatization of the former.

ANN'S VERSION OF THE STORY

At the time Ann brought in the story of "Hansel and Gretel" to the drama therapy training group, I asked her which character she most identified with. She named Hansel:

> He was the person who had to take care of any emergency, and in this story, life-and-death issues. I am the oldest child of five and grew up with an alcoholic father. I could clearly identify with this hero role.

Thus began Ann's dramatic exploration of the role of hero as rescuer who used her charms, wit, and courage to save her father from his murderous feelings. To illustrate this point, she told the following story:

> *In the early 1970s, a young girl of 9 was again awakened from her sleep by a strange noise. She got out of bed and proceeded cautiously toward the kitchen. There was her father, as before, with his back turned. He was sharpening a knife. The sound of the blade against the squeaky wheels of an old can opener frightened her. It was 3 A.M. She summoned all her courage this time.*
> *What are you doing? she asked.*
> *You think I'm gonna kill you, don't you? replied the startled father.*
> *No, no, of course not, said the young girl.*
> *Her tone became lighter. She calmed him in the jokey, seductive manner she had by this time mastered when her father had been drinking. He was dangerous and needed to be rescued from himself. She knew this better than anyone, because she had chosen to take on the role of the rescuer.*

In enacting the heroic role of Hansel and working with others in the group who had chosen their own identified roles, Ann was able to work through that moment of terror in the kitchen, transforming her hero role from that of one who rescued the father by denying her own needs to that of one who could rescue herself by expressing those needs.

Ann first told the story of "Hansel and Gretel" to the group. Following the storytelling, members of the group chose characters with whom they identified and proceeded to dramatize the story. The experience lasted 3 hours. In the weeks following the therapeutic story dramatization, Ann was able to relate the fiction to her real-life experience. In describing the process, I include some of Ann's subsequent reflections.

Ann began the story as follows:

A widower, with two children, had remarried. They were all very poor, and the stepmother convinced the father to send the children out into the forest to die, so that they could eat The father resisted, but then gave in to the sinister logic of his wife late one night Unbeknownst to them, they are overheard by Hansel and Gretel. Hansel convinces Gretel not to be afraid. He will save them.

Ann reflected upon the fact that she would often stay awake at night to watch over her family. She often sat up with her inebriated father and listened to his litany of fears and anxieties. Said Ann later:

> I was making sure he was OK and that the rest of the family was protected from him. When within the drama we played Hansel and Gretel overhearing their parents, I felt how terrified Hansel was, and then how terrified I must have been. But because he felt that his role was to take care of Gretel, he had no other option but to put his fear away and go on.

In her version of the story, Ann initially conceived of Hansel as a martyr who must sacrifice himself so that others will survive. Her version of Hansel was complex, as she also saw him as an adolescent rebel, one who rejects the oppressive and unreasonable demands of the parents. The roles of martyr and rebel mirror Ann's own experience of adolescence, when she both martyred herself to save her family and rebelled against their oppressive diet to journey into the world outside for sexual and spiritual sustenance.

Ann conceived of her martyr role as a rebel willing to die for a cause. The cause, however, was to maintain the integrity of the dysfunctional family: the sickness and anger of the father, the total denial of the mother, the victimization of the children. Thus, this rebel/martyr role caused Ann much ambivalence. If only she could die for a more virtuous cause—if only she could live by truly rebelling and rejecting the family sickness—then she could truly feed herself.

Adding further to the ambivalence, Ann saw Hansel the martyr as resentful, a quality very unlike that of the classic martyr, who bears a cross proudly. In Ann's version, Hansel feels resentful toward Gretel for having to take care of her, and toward the father for having given in to the mother's sinister plan of removing the children. Such feelings echo Ann's resentments toward her real-life siblings and father.

Her version of the fairy tale continued:

When they are first sent into the woods, Hansel is clever and drops a trail of white stones behind them. He and Gretel follow the trail illuminated by moonlight back home. But he is unable to rest The parents, hav-

ing rejected the children once, will surely try again. He was bothered by the fact that he didn't hear their scheming the next time. Could he have been sleeping? When they were again taken to the woods, he left a trail of bread crumbs. When he discovered that the birds had eaten the crumbs, he was really freaked out He had messed up. He was an imperfect hero, frustrated and embarrassed, overwhelmed.

At this point in Ann's account, imperfections begin to appear in the persona of Hansel. The mask of the hero as rescuer begins to crack. Hansel foolishly believes that food, represented by bread crumbs, is an effective substitute for the permanence and neutrality of stones. Ann referred to stones as being safe, whereas food is false security— that which appears to nourish but, in fact, leaves one empty. Even the kind of food used, bread crumbs, represents a meal fit only for beggars. Faced with his mistake, Ann's version of Hansel feels his heroic role slip away. He becomes a simpleton, ignorant of alternative solutions, and a lost one, humiliated and purposeless.

Such had been the state of affairs when Ann's heroic efforts to save the members of her family failed totally. They too quickly gobbled up the few crumbs she tried to throw them like a lifeline. Aware that she could no longer lead her family back home, she too lost her purpose.

Ann continued:

Hansel and Gretel wander in the forest until they come to a clearing. They look up and see a gingerbread house and begin to eat the sweets from the roof. A good witch appears and invites them in. When inside the house, the good witch turns into a bad witch and threatens to eat the children.

Hansel is tricked; according to Ann, this is what he expects as punishment for being imperfect. The message for Ann seems to be this: Lose the way for the family, abrogate the rescuer role, and all that appears good will upon closer examination become evil. In the role of the lost one, Ann herself, like Hansel, felt hopeless. Asking for help is dangerous, because the helper is actually a deceiver who offers food only as a trap to devour the hungry one.

Ann identified her mother as a good witch who seduced her into believing that she had the power to rescue the father and save the family. When the father would drink, he often became physically abusive; in pain and fear, Ann would go to her mother for help. When approached, however, her mother would transform herself into the bad witch and deny the chaos, often accusing Ann of flights of fancy. Through her denial, the nourishing mother consumed her daughter.

The story proceeded:

After Hansel was captured, he had no options. He just let things go on. The witch tried to fatten him up by locking him in a cage and stuffing him full of food. He tried to pretend he was not getting fat by sticking a skinny stick through the bars of the cage for the wicked witch to feel.

Ann had been struggling with her role of eater for some years, taking on weight and shedding it, filling up and emptying herself repeatedly. The fattening of Hansel reflected Ann's sense of getting fat on resentment and ambivalence. Like Hansel she too sat in a kind of psychic cage, eating to cover up her frustration with the rescuer role. For all the world to see, she displayed a skinny stick, a false image of a happy, skinny woman. In assuring the others that she was OK, she hoped to assure herself. Her ploy worked, at least to the extent that many of the others accepted the false image. Yet she lived in a self-deception, unable to lift the weight of her family from her imprisoned body.

Anne went on:

When Gretel finally saved them by killing the witch, Hansel was almost numb. He had no desire to go home, but he enjoyed the way home, a sort of limbo from all his problems.

Since moving from her parents' house, Ann had lived in 15 different homes. She had been unable to settle down for fear of repeating the domestic life she had experienced with her parents and siblings. Each move held the hope of finally discovering a safe house; Ann enjoyed the process of moving toward home. But in reality each move signaled a replay of the past. Thus, the rescuer role played by Gretel reflected an ambivalent reaction within Ann: Hansel was free and not free at the same time.

Ann continued:

When they arrived home, the father was waiting without the mother (she had died) and really was glad to see the children. They went to sleep. Hansel lay awake and steamed.

With the mother's death, a significant offstage act, Hansel now has the father all to himself. What will he do? Within the group, I noted that Ann stood at a crossroads at this point. She was clearly agitated. What would she do? To be or not to be? I asked her to improvise her own ending. She responded directly:

Hansel and Gretel arrived home and the father was very glad to see them. They went to sleep. Hansel got up in the middle of the night and killed his father. And Hansel and Gretel lived happily ever after.

ANN AND JANET:
LEVELS OF DRAMATIC INTERACTIONS

Within the group drama therapy process, Ann first told her version of the story, and then enacted it with others in their chosen roles as Gretel, Father, Mother, Good Witch, Bad Witch, Gingerbread House (or Goody House, as the group member playing the role called it), and the Way Home. Upon completing the enactment, Ann felt a sense of relief, even though she expressed a fear of the others' judgment for resolving the story so violently. She was especially concerned about the reaction of Janet, the woman playing Hansel's father, claiming:

> I feel like I was very honest with my feelings, but living in the resentment almost killed off the person playing the father.

I wondered which father she was talking about. Was Ann's central concern about "killing" Janet? If so, what did that mean? Janet was the most vulnerable member of the group, recently a victim of a brutal rape. Although not the daughter of a dysfunctional father, Janet grew up with a very powerful yet distant father, who was involved in moral causes that kept him away from home.

Ann recalled an early experience in the group. All had brought in objects from home and scattered them around the room. They were asked to choose several objects to play with and to begin to relate to others in the group through the objects. One person had brought in a real switchblade knife. This was the only unsafe object present, and most avoided playing with it; Janet was the one exception. In wielding the unsafe object, she frightened several in the group, especially Ann. In the play, Ann found herself back in the kitchen as a little girl, trying to find a way to neutralize the overwhelming power of her drunken father, sitting with his back turned, sharpening a kitchen knife. In her play, spontaneously, Ann found a way to neutralize her fears: She reached into her purse and pulled out her diaphragm. The image released a lot of laughter and transformed the moment of fear to that of safety. This time Ann seemed to be saying: It's all fun; no one is going to get hurt; the contraceptive is mightier than the sword.

In reflecting upon her drama of Hansel and Gretel, Ann recognized the connection between Janet, who played the father in the story, and her own father in the kitchen. Both embodied the paradoxical qualities of the victim and the victimizer. In working through her ambivalences, Ann was able to conceive of the father as a role taken on from her own father. As she came to see it, the dysfunctional father role must be symbolically killed in order for more functional ones to live.

Ann's relationship to Janet within the context of the dramatization points to the complexity of dramatic role interactions, which exist on four levels: theatrical, archetypal, transferential, and everyday.*

The theatrical level concerns the relationship between actors and their roles or one role and another within the dramatization. On the theatrical level in this case, there were the following interactions:

1. Ann in relation to Hansel.
2. Hansel in relation to Hansel's father.
3. Janet in relation to Hansel's father.
4. Hansel's father in relation to Hansel.
5. Hansel or Hansel's father in relation to any other character(s) in the dramatization.

The archetypal level is that of one role type in relation to another. That role type can be expressed as fictional or nonfictional. At the archetypal level in this instance, there were the following interactions:

1. Rescuer/hero in relation to father.
2. Son/daughter in relation to father.
3. Victimizer in relation to victim.

The transferential level is one in which the fictional character becomes symbolic of a significant relationship in the actor's everyday life. In relating to the significant other, the actor attempts to work

---

*In a discussion of his structural role model, Johnson (1981) offers a somewhat similar scheme, describing four levels of dramatic interaction between two people in an improvisation:

a. Impersonal: the relationship between two enacted roles (e.g., that of Hansel and Hansel's father).
b. Intrapersonal: the relationship between each person and his own role (e.g., that between Ann and Hansel, Janet and Hansel's father).
c. Extrapersonal: the relationship between each person and the other person's role (e.g., that between Ann and Hansel's father, Janet and Hansel).
d. Interpersonal: the relationship between the two individuals (e.g., that between Ann and Janet).

Johnson's description of his model is part of an article about the schizophrenic condition; accordingly, he expresses concerns about boundary confusions and helping clients maintain distinctions between one role and another on theatrical, transferential, and everyday levels.

through a condition stimulated in the fictional context. Examples in this case included the following:

1. Ann in relation to Hansel's father.
2. Janet in relation to Hansel.
3. Janet in relation to Hansel's father.

Finally, at the nonfictional level of everyday experience, an actual relationship takes place outside the context of theatrical role playing. In this case it involved the following:

1. Ann in relation to Janet.
2. Janet in relation to Ann.

In understanding Ann's statement above concerning her homicidal feelings, we need to consider the possibility of all four levels. Thus, the father she spoke about may have been theatrical, archetypal, transferential, or nonfictional. Or it may have been that Ann's "father" existed on all levels, and Ann's struggle became one of locating that father role wherever it might exist, then working it through in such a way that it became functional within her role system. The same process, if effective, applied to Janet and all others within the group who interacted with Ann in and out of role. Furthermore, it applies to all roles that are invoked, named, and worked through in any therapeutic dramatization.

FICTION AND NONFICTION: ANN'S SUBSEQUENT WORK

Following the storytelling and enactment, Ann took a step back from the theatrical level and began to make connections between fictional and nonfictional roles. In speaking of these roles, she addressed their archetypal substance as she related them to her everyday experiences. She focused first on the role of murderer, which she characterized as the most frightening one within her role system. She reflected upon the past:

When I was 6, I was playing house (my favorite game) in the backyard of Sally B., and Sally would not do what I told her to do. Little Ann got so mad that she threw a spoon in Sally's eye. It missed, but cut her face so bad that she had to get stitches. Little Ann was completely frozen and terrified. The anger was howling. I am powerful enough to hurt and kill. I thought I would never live this trauma down. The guilt of acting on the anger was unbelievable and powerful. I went home and lied to my mother that I did not mean to throw the spoon at Sally. I think my mother wanted to believe this. But I knew ever since that if I show how angry I get, I will never, ever be able to protect people from this. I will kill them.

About a year later, Sally's sister, Mary, knocked me down and pushed all my baby teeth back in my head. This was awful, but I remember thinking that I deserved it My mother ran into Mrs. B. many years later, and she said that Sally still had a scar from the accident My mother said that Mary got back at me for that scar. So even today, someone is walking around with scars of my anger.

The murderer part of Ann, then, is the other side of the rescuer, more akin to the rebel who rejects the restraints of a suffocating family life. Ann recognized the extreme quality of the murderer archetype. It functioned for her, on the one hand, as a danger signal, reminding her not to fully abandon the rescuer role, but rather to use it as a means of rescuing herself from the fear of hurting others. On the other hand, the murderer role functioned to provide Ann with the impetus to act—on an intrapsychic level by killing off her passive, self-destructive, masochistic tendencies, and on an interpersonal level by striking back at those attempting to stifle her journey toward a functional role system.

Ann presented another version of the rescuer–murderer dyad in speaking of the tension between two related archetypes of savior and malcontent. For Ann, the savior is one who, like the prototypical Christ, attempts to rescue others. But Ann also described the savior as a kind of fool who fails in his messianic attempts by tripping over his own piety. The savior role is a bit embarrassing, and in its failure invokes a counterpart, the malcontent.

The malcontent is an angry, sometimes rageful role that subsists on all the perceived ills of a world. But, as in the case of the savior, Ann conceived of this role in a complex way. The malcontent is most often a hidden role, disguised in a pleasant, skinny, stick-like demeanor. The danger in this role is that it may become too overwhelming, leading to that of the murderer. Although more manageable, it functioned to steer Ann clear of her tendency to take her Christ-like roles too seriously. When in balance, the savior and the malcontent role allowed Ann to take care of herself. They further allowed her to view her need to help others with a critical eye, and to pull back after falling into old family patterns.

Ann viewed both the father and mother roles negatively. She added further information about the father role, which she conceived as cowardly, impotent, and ineffectual, ever complying with the mother part, which is powerful, demanding, and selfish. Ann saw the former role as keeping her safe from having to make decisions or take any responsibility for her actions, and the latter role as a dark version of the murderer, wishing everyone dead so that it may live.

Thus, the murderous mother exerts a greater psychic power than the murderous father. This mother role would devour all other roles if it could, breaking down the integrity of the role system. This murderous mother would withhold nurturance or, most heinously, assume the archetypal power of Medea, murdering her children and serving them up for dinner. As an introject, the role of murderous mother served Ann negatively, keeping her locked into a starvation mentality—a need to deprive herself of emotional sustenance and to control other parts of her role system that might try to smuggle in healthy foods.

Ann noted that the mother holds two other roles within her dominion: that of food and that of home. Ann saw food as a wish fulfillment, a desire to be nurtured and loved. Yet in the search for such psychic sustenance, Ann felt ambivalent, simultaneously famished and full. Like Kafka's hunger artist, she could not seem to find the right food, and thus abused that which was available. The food role kept her in an existential state of guilt and, at times, despair. In that she saw the mother roles as trying to starve her, the food role adhered to the mother complex.

Home was also an ambivalent image for Ann. In reflecting upon it as a role, she called it hell, the place of overwhelming role ambivalence. The role of home served Ann not as a secure place, but as a trap. Only the way home offered a psychic alternative, a path, a process holding forth the promise of security built apart from the mother. As a role, the way home was supported by the white stones—beautiful pieces of nature, permanent and trustworthy, illuminating the way home and providing a safe path.

The negative female role is further delineated in the personae of the good and bad witches. Ann saw the good witch as manipulative and seductive, like the mother, locked into a power struggle that she must win. As an intrapsychic role, it functioned to deceive other parts of Ann, especially those in need of nurturance. The bad witch is simply immoral, making no attempts at concealing her desires. Her need is to do evil, and she will pursue those ends vigorously. This part of Ann appeared in her rebellious actions, providing a good foil for the part of her that pretended to be innocent and compliant.

Finally, Ann spoke of the effects of the brother and sister roles—those innocents, orphans, victims, and wise children who are able ultimately to outsmart the evils of the parents and the demonic witches, asserting a more adult, experienced warrior quality. Gretel, as sister, reflects the needy yet wise feminine part of Ann. This part served her, finally, in solving baffling problems through wisdom, patience, and an ability to perform well under difficult circumstances.

The sister role well complements the brother role, exemplified in Hansel, who is clever and strong but tends to break down when confronted with his imperfections. In the boy role, Ann saw herself as aggressive and domineering, capable of being a buddy and peer to men. The masculine and feminine roles together, like the interplay of Hansel and Gretel, served Ann in a liberating way. Gretel kills an image of the mother in the persona of the witch. Hansel kills the father; like Hamlet, he has finally acted to remove the object of his resentment. In murdering the murderer, Ann symbolically resolved Hamlet's famous ambivalence. She chose her own being, rejecting self-slaughter as an alternative. Having taken on qualities of both Hansel and Gretel, Ann was ready to forge out on her own, sexually and spiritually.

The murderous father wielding a knife still loomed in Ann's psyche as a fearful image that surfaced from time to time in transferential relationships, such as that with Janet mentioned above. But the destructive power of the inner father was significantly diminished. And, in fact, Ann was able to establish a committed relationship with an older man. With the wisdom and strength of both young warrior roles, Ann would make a home for herself apart from her father and mother, both of whom she had symbolically murdered. She would continue to move beyond her roles of rescuer and martyr, and to find further ways to assume that of the hero, who journeys home after slaying the dreaded dragon with the expectation of finding a nourishing meal on the table. Aware of her transferences and of the functions of her theatrical roles, Ann could now build a rich existence among her archetypal and everyday roles.

WORK BY OTHER GROUP MEMBERS

Ann was the central figure in this drama therapy experience. In many ways, the other members of the group supported Ann in her exploration of the Hansel role. However, the experience very much concerned the full group, and all members were encouraged to work through their own issues embodied in their chosen roles. The other roles chosen, as mentioned above, included Gretel, the Mother, the Father, the Good Witch (which the client playing the role called "the saddest delusion"), the Bad Witch, the Gingerbread House (or Goody House), and the Way Home.

Following a lengthy discussion reflecting upon the experience and attempting to uncover some connections between the roles and the role players, I asked all members of the group to revise the story from the point of view of their chosen characters. The following was told by Dora, who took on the role of Gretel. Dora worked often within the archetypal level of role enactment, attempting to discover those universal forms that reflected her combined moral and cultural concerns. She called her story "Gretel and Hansel":

Once upon a time a young girl named Gretel lived with her woodcutter father, her mean mother, and her loving brother, Hansel. While Gretel's father loved his children, the mother was incapable of loving and made the children work hard around the house. Gretel was happy for the father's love, but took her consolation from her closeness with Hansel. Hansel loved to take care of Gretel, which she would allow and enjoy. Really, though, Gretel was always the more resourceful of the two.

One night Gretel and Hansel overheard the parents planning a way to leave the children in the woods. Hansel decided he would gather stones to find their way back. Gretel was comforted by this and they fell asleep. The next day, the family journeyed to the woods, whereupon Hansel dropped his stones. Sure enough, the children were left in the woods, and as the moon rose over the landscape, the children followed the reflected light of the moon in the white pebbles. This was a sign that the children would ultimately be guided home by the feminine principle, represented by the moon. Upon reaching their home, the mother screamed and yelled, and the father expressed his happiness with the children's return. The children were sent to their rooms to clean, however, as the mother's wish always prevailed. Gretel knew and accepted this, happy that Hansel had to clean his room too, and that she was not alone.

The children overheard the same conversation to abandon them in the woods. This time Hansel told Gretel not to worry, that he would throw bread crumbs to find the trail home. Gretel knew something did not feel right about this, but had a hard time telling her brother that she knew his solutions were lame. But after all, his last solution had worked. It was just easier to depend upon him and stroke his ego, and be taken care of.

The next day, they were abandoned in the woods again, and when the moon rose to light the path home, the bread crumbs had been eaten up by birds. Gretel and Hansel searched and searched for the proper trail. At one point Gretel had a strong feeling for the way home. But she followed Hansel's directions instead, those that took them to the Gingerbread House. So happy to see something delicious to eat, Gretel and Hansel set about devouring the house, despite its protestations. Soon an old woman poked her head out of the house, inviting them in to comfort. Upon entering the house, a mean witch appeared, separated Gretel and Hansel, and threw Hansel into a cage to fatten up for a meal. Gretel was totally freaked out She was actually angry at Hansel for leaving her, but felt guilty for being angry at him. After all, he was to be dinner.

The witch forced Gretel to cook and clean, while Gretel frantically searched for a way to save her brother. No doubt about it, she had to come up with the solutions this time or lose him forever in the most hideous manner. As the witch was ready to place Hansel in the oven, Gretel said she never liked her brother anyway and she would prepare the oven for him. She pretended that the pilot light went out, and when the witch went inside the oven to light it, Gretel pushed her in with a triumphant rebel yell.

Gretel and Hansel ran out of the house and found the way home that Gretel had glimpsed earlier. Upon reaching home, the father tearfully and happily greeted his beloved children and told them of their mother's death. Everyone was glad she was dead. Gretel and Hansel went off to bed. Gretel was happy to be home with Hansel and her loving father, but became aware of a growing dissatisfaction within Hansel. Gretel knew she could now rely on herself, maybe tell her brother when he was bothering her and let herself be separate from him so that he can work out his own problems. She learned that you don't have to be fused to another to be close and happy, that when you are separate you can really be authentically closer.

In this example, Dora conceived of Gretel as hero. Her journey was one through the complexity and ambivalences of gender. Hers was a feminist struggle for power, beginning by deferring to the wisdom and strength of the male figures and ending with the discovery of her own power as a wise, strong, and moral woman. At the end, Dora as Gretel chose a connected separateness, serving her needs for both independence and interdependence. Her family roles were in order: The father is loving and presumably forgiven for his cowardice in the face of his wife; the mean, murderous mother and witch are dead; and the loving brother, although dissatisfied (with the father? with the fact that his sister was the hero and not he?), is safely tucked in bed, ready to be separated from. In de-roling from Gretel, Dora recognized this family configuration as an ideal.

Reflecting upon the images of women represented in the story, Dora saw two homes—that of Hansel and Gretel and the Gingerbread House, presided over by brutal mother figures. Both women serve negative functions. The positive feminine model appears in the persona of the moon, whose purpose is to illuminate the way home. Thus, the positive feminine role points one in the direction home, providing the process, the illumination, the way. In struggling against the dark, devouring mother within herself, Dora heroically looked for the appropriate paths in her life that would lead her to her personal strength and social relatedness. She recognized that sometimes along the way she would need to take on the power of both the murderer and rescuer roles, in order to liberate herself from the constraints of cowardly and defeated men, selfish and hungry women and the parts of her personality generating those qualities. In order to put her domestic roles fully in order, Dora saw that she must first take the hero's journey into the dark woods of the psyche.

For much of the group experience, Connie had difficulty with Dora, identifying her as her jealous sister. At the beginning of the group process, she had no awareness of the transferential level that occurred whenever she interacted with Dora. Like Ann, Connie came from an alcoholic family; through her work in a self-help group called Adult Children of Alcoholics, she began to examine her role as codependent, which serves to enable family members to stay in their dysfunctional roles, even as the codependent attempts to rescue them (see McFarland & Baker-Baumann, 1989).

In many ways, Connie's family history resembled that of Cinderella. Like Cinderella, her beauty far surpassed that of her jealous sister; yet she worked for the family, picking up the cinders of their repressed rage, trying to hold things together. To do that, like Cinderella, she needed to be the good girl, the perfectionist, the humble one. As an adult, she escaped the drabness of her dysfunctional family by becoming a successful commercial actress. This fact further inflamed her sister's jealousy.

Since this was the story of Hansel and Gretel, Connie felt somewhat removed from the given cast of characters. She felt drawn, however, to the Gingerbread House. When addressing the question of why she chose the role, she responded:

> I had no idea why as we began the enactment. At first I was the nurturing house, anxious to feed the poor children, but after a while I became hurt by their seeming greediness and was overwhelmed by self-pity. This self-pity turned to anger, which was expressed but was ignored by Hansel and Gretel. To admit this is difficult, because this "Goody House" as I called it, is a metaphor for my life as the hero in an alcoholic family. I'd followed the exact same pattern, giving too much of myself and then feeling depleted, without being consciously aware of it.

For Connie, an understanding of the Goody House role allowed her to see how easily the hero/rescuer role can be transformed into that of the victim. In her work toward reconstructing her role system, she had slowly allowed the victim role to disengage from the rescuer. The Goody House part of her was still alluring and sweet, yet inside was something far greater than a murderous and ravenous old hag. Inside the house of beauty, there were also strength and wisdom. The part of Connie that was like Cinderella got her prince (i.e., got her needs met), but not by waiting passively for a man to knock on her door with a glass slipper. This alternative Cinderella part of Connie believed that she must actively pursue her fantasies and move on with her journey, even though some along the way would try to eat her up. When that happened and the self-pitying victim emerged, Connie attempted to catch herself and recognize her right to continue unencumbered.

Toward the end of the training group, Connie recognized her transference onto Dora. In making the separation between her jealous sister, who continued to belittle her, and Dora, who in reality supported Connie's heroic search, Connie was able to resolve her transference.

A fourth group member, Julia, played the role of the children's mother. Like Ann and Connie, she was the daughter of an alcoholic father. Julia came from a large family where she took on the maternal, nurturing role to her siblings. Yet in many ways, Julia saw herself as the other side of the coin—a cold, evil mother who really wanted unlimited power over others. In revising the Hansel and Gretel tale, she created a story entitled "The Mother Who Was Born without a Heart":

Once upon a time there lived an empty shell of a person. She appeared to be a woman; she had breasts and wore a skirt, and so she was. She had the exteriors, hence others saw her as a female, but the woman felt nothing inside. No feelings, warmth, or other feminine sensations; no sexual feelings; just empty and barren.

A man came by one day and saw her as a woman and made his bed with her. The man had many feelings inside, but he felt empty whenever he was inside of this woman. The woman conceived two children. They grew inside of her, but she still felt nothing. She spit them out with relief. She could make no milk to feed these babies. The father seemed to love the babies. This made the woman tense. It always gave her a headache. Headaches were the only feelings she had. She could also feel the pain when she mutilated herself. Many times she would chew her fingers or place the hot iron on her leg. The burning sensation made her feel alive. The woman liked to kill insects and small animals. She would grit her teeth tightly together and lock her jaw firmly while she performed these rituals. This seemed to relieve some pressure in her head.

The woman's husband was often depressed and worked very little. The woman kept a very neat and orderly house. She wanted everything in order, but it was very messy. Her kids were especially messy. They whimpered a lot and often tried to crawl into her lap for comfort, wrinkling her skirt or messing up the well-made bed. This would only give the woman a headache, and she'd need to kill another small animal.

She took pleasure in depriving her children, forcing them to skip meals, interrupting their games with chores. She made them her slaves. She could only feel a relief of headache pressure if they were following her orders. Then everything felt clean and neat. As the children became older, they be-

came difficult to manage, and it made the woman very uncomfortable. She feared losing all control and wanted them out of her life.

Her husband, who was always easily manipulated by the woman, was convinced to dump the two children in the woods. The woman was sure that the only way she could continue was without them. So he did take them away. When he returned without them, the woman felt so relieved that she killed five small animals by boiling them alive. She laughed and laughed and laughed until suddenly she became aware of her own eerie laugh echoing inside of a hollow self. She felt the empty, barren, barrel-like inside begin to widen and consume her entire being. This terrorized the woman. Her emptiness began to swallow her alive.

In desperation, the lost woman flung herself into the boiling pot with the small animals. The boiling water engulfed her body and she felt great relief. She lay in the boiling pot—floating. Her body began to swell and puff like a piece of pasta. She puffed all out, and her headache subsided. Her insides began to blister, and each blister began to drip. Drip tears. The blisters oozed and oozed tears, and finally tears began to leak from the woman's eyes and she felt total bliss. Just before the calm of death overtook the parboiled woman, a smile came over her face, and she secretly wished her children and husband well.

The qualities of this mother are portrayed in a Gothic style reminiscent of Jacobean revenge tragedies, such as *The Duchess of Malfi* and *The White Devil*, which are studies in the excesses and cruelties committed in the pursuit of power. This mother has only the trappings of femininity—breasts and skirt—but is otherwise asexual and demonic. She withholds food and love, and can only experience things of the heart through extreme forms of sadism and masochism.

This is a Dionysian woman, like Agave from *The Bacchae*, who brutally murders her son while under the spell of Dionysus, and Medea, who is capable of destroying and mutilating her children. She is a tyrant, whose need for power has no limits. She is both murderer and suicide whose actions, finally, serve a therapeutic purpose: to help her acquire the precious thing she was always deprived of—her heart, her ability to feel. In the end, she finds her heart, but pays dearly for it with her life.

For Julia, the inner role of the heartless woman functioned to hide the helpless, needy child. Julia described that child as sad and rageful because her needs for nurturance were never met by her parents. Julia, too, had an inner victim part that must remain hidden for fear of being further neglected and abused.

The role of the heartless mother came up with regularity in Julia's dramas. It was a reminder not only to pay more attention to the needy child, but also to find a way to more fully express the adult sexual woman, with heart and head intact. Julia's search, then, concerned a means to allow the vulnerable child part of herself to live without denying the potentially overwhelming power of the adult woman. In reflecting upon the story of the heartless woman, she recognized yet again her need to live in the ambivalence of sex and death, pain and pleasure, innocence and experience, powerful and overpowering feelings, child and woman.

After a year of work, the group had became quite cohesive for the most part. By the time "Hansel and Gretel" was dramatized, many of the dynamics had already been established. Ann, Connie, and Julia in many ways played similar roles within the group. All had been both rescuers and victims of their dysfunctional families, and they carried that role ambivalence with them into the group. Although they were different in quality—Ann facing the world with the "skinny stick," good-girl persona; Connie going beyond appearance to offer good things to needy people; and Julia, in a reversal of the good-girl image, raging against those who needed her nurturance—all tended to galvanize the group and take responsibility for its well-being. In their different ways, they felt responsible for the forces that threatened the integrity of the group: those of jealousy, authority, and powerlessness.

Dora played out her quest for power independently, even while, like the Gretel of her story, she sought out affiliation with her group sisters. In fact, taking their cue from the story, most group members attempted to recreate a family of close and supportive siblings who needed each other in order to survive, as they were put out in the harsh world by fathers and mothers of questionable moral authority. In finally de-roling at the end of the experience, most were able to see these dynamics and understand how their roles contributed to this society of peers.

One exception was Janet in the role of Hansel's father. As noted above, Ann felt that her dramatic act of killing the father frightened Janet, who in fact stopped coming to the group for several weeks thereafter. Her return was sporadic, after which she withdrew from the group for a time. This was not Janet's family. She was from a more privileged socioeconomic background than the others, used to the company of wealthy and powerful people. But even so, there were ambivalences: A minority-group member herself, she worked with the disenfranchised. Although privileged, she bore the traumatic scars of the victim of rape. Even though she had been an active and integral part of the group for some months, her style of role playing was underdistanced—too real and too close to the edge. The story of Hansel and Gretel, focusing upon issues of victimization was too reflective of Janet's real-life dilemma. And the other group members, though well aware of Janet's recent history, could not fully support her within the story dramatization: She played out the fictional roles of deceiver and victimizer, and they felt obliged to respond in role. They were, for the most part, playing within a theatrical context. Janet kept slipping too often into the transferential and everyday ones, which became too difficult to bear as they restimulated her abuse.

The fate of the father in the story was hotly contested. Some, like Ann, wished to punish his weakness. Others, like Dora, wished to forgive not only the father, but also the weak part of the psyche that tends to cave in to the demands of villains. Janet, in the role of father, needed distance from the drama and the overwhelming ambivalences she was feeling on a personal level. She was simply too exposed and too merged with the role of victim. Whether facing the knife or wielding the knife, her drama was too real. In her post-traumatic state, she had little ability to view the connection between the fictional and the everyday. Neither the group nor I as the leader was able to help her journey forth beyond the reality of the crisis or find her way back home from the crisis.

In retrospect, Janet needed more time in individual therapy. And within the group, she needed safer roles. Could we have replayed the story of Hansel and Gretel, we might have recognized the inappropriateness of the father role or of the group process in general for Janet. In many ways, Janet left the group in the role thrust upon her by Ann—that of unwilling, passive accomplice, a victim who meant to do good. When she left, she resumed her slow process of healing within a supportive family network. In her struggle with post-traumatic stress disorder, she searched for the strength of the survivor who can endure in the face of desperate circumstances, and the warrior who, like Hansel and Gretel, can defeat the dreaded demons and return home, marked but intact.

For many people, that safe road home was once upon a time a fairy-tale world taken on in childhood. For functional adults, the way back home is the path that is simultaneously fairy tale and bald reality: the ideal roles promised by our parents, and the real ones encountered as those promises are broken by many symbolic parents. To be victim and not to be victim, to venture out on an unsafe journey and to return to a safe home—that was the essential story of Hansel and Gretel played out by this drama therapy group.

IMPLICATIONS OF THE ROLE
METHOD FOR DIAGNOSIS

There have been few attempts to develop means of diagnosing clients purely from a drama therapy perspective. Existing approaches by drama therapists are based primarily on two models: psychoanalysis and psychological development. Irwin (Irwin, 1985; Irwin & Shapiro, 1975) and Portner (Irwin & Malloy, 1975; Portner, 1981) have discussed the use of a puppetry interview for both the individual client and the family group, whereby participants are asked to speak improvisationally with or through hand puppets. In the case of family therapy, a basket containing different puppets is offered to the family. The members choose which ones they feel drawn to and present a spontaneous puppet show. The actual psychodynamics are assessed by the therapist as a means of guiding further treatment. Irwin and Portner base their approach on a psychoanalytic model and apply psychoanalytical criteria to their assessment. In assessing their clients, the researchers examine both the content and form of the puppet play.

Johnson (1988) has devised a diagnostic method based on improvisation, called the "diagnostic role-playing test." In its two versions, clients are either given a list of five social roles and asked to play them out, or simply instructed to play out the roles of three beings of their own choice. In both instances, Johnson applies criteria garnered from his developmental approach, which is derived from both developmental psychology and object relations theory (Johnson, 1991). Johnson's criteria include the following:

1. Structure of space, tasks, and roles in a scene.
2. Media of representation (sound, movement, image, word) used in a scene.
3. Complexity of characters and settings.
4. Interactions among characters.
5. Forms and degrees of affect.

When the role method is applied to diagnosis, the following criteria can serve to help assess the initial functioning of a client:

1. Ability to invoke and name roles.
2. Number of roles invoked and named.
3. Ability to attribute qualities to the roles.
4. Ability to delineate alternative qualities or subroles.
5. Ability to perceive the function of role as role.
6. Style of role playing and aesthetic distance present in role playing.
7. Ability to relate the fictional role to everyday life.

In proceeding diagnostically through the role method, the therapist generally asks clients first to tell a story, and then to name the roles within the story, specifying their qualities and alternative qualities, functions, and connections to their everyday lives. The therapist also notes the style of role playing employed, with its concomitant degree of affect and/or cognition. The storytelling process can be done individually or in a small group such as a family; in the latter case, the therapist focuses not only upon the role qualities, functions, and styles, but also upon the dynamic interactions that occur in the collaborative creation of the story.

If a client requires a less verbal test, the therapist can work through either movement or sandplay. The movement approach has been described to some extent in Chapter Three. It involves asking a client or small group to move around the room, focus upon one body part, extend that body part out into space, and allow a character to emerge. A discussion follows according to the given diagnostic criteria.

The sandplay approach involves the use of miniature objects (e.g., people, animals, structures, and vehicles provided by the therapist), which the client arranges in picture form within a rectangular sand-tray, approximately 2 feet by 4 feet. Generally sandplay is practiced individually, as described in regard to Michael in Chapter Four, but it can also occur with two or perhaps three people working collaboratively in creating a sand picture. Following the creation of the picture, a story based upon the content can be told, or the therapist can move directly to a discussion of the roles created in the sandtray.

In looking at the first criterion, ability to invoke and name roles, clients can be diagnosed on a 3-point continuum. The lowest end, 1, represents clients who are unable to invoke a role. The middle, 2, indicates the ability to invoke a role but not to name it. The highest point, 3, indicates the ability both to invoke a single role and to give it a name.

The next criterion, number of roles invoked and named, can be rated according to quantity, the low ends corresponding to the 3 points above. The next point, 4, indicates those able to invoke and name several (up to three) roles. At the high end are those able to invoke and name more than three roles. Such a scale may be difficult to interpret, however, in that some techniques (e.g., the movement exercise) call for the invocation and naming of a single role, whereas others (e.g., storytelling and sandplay) call for multiple roles. The clients who are able to invoke and name the most roles, then, are not necessarily the ones who perform at the highest level. In some cases, such clients may be performing dysfunctionally (i.e., if they have been specifically asked to invoke a single role). Generally speaking, dysfunctional clients are those who are incapable of invoking and naming any roles, or those who invoke and name too many or too few roles. Clients who are able to invoke and name a number of roles appropriate to a given task are performing within the normal range.

In terms of quality of roles, the therapist asks the client following the enactment to generally discuss the qualities or attributes of the roles specified. Some clients may need more specific instructions, in which case the therapist offers a range of qualities within one or more of the following domains:

1. Physical (e.g., from strong to weak, healthy to sick, gay to straight, young to old, beautiful to average to ugly).
2. Cognitive (e.g., from simple to complex, ignorant to wise, ambivalent to dogmatic).
3. Moral (e.g., from innocent to deceptive, victimized to victimizing, moral to immoral, gregarious to miserly, cowardly to brave).
4. Emotional (e.g., from angry to peaceful, hating to loving, lifeless to ecstatic).
5. Social (e.g., from family-oriented to rebellious, bourgeois to aristocratic, poor to rich, alienated to social).
6. Political (e.g., from conservative to radical, authoritarian to democratic).
7. Spiritual (e.g., from atheistic to orthodox, heroic to nihilistic, Dionysian to Apollonian).
8. Aesthetic (e.g., from creative to uncreative, idealistic to realistic).

Clients responding within the normal range are those able to identify at least three qualitative categories. For example, in specifying the qualities of a female role called Pious, a client may speak of the character's physical appearance, as well as her strong attachment to the family and to an orthodox religious faith. At the low end of the scale are the clients unable to attribute any qualities at all to the role. Those able to specify one or a limited number are also functioning at a relatively low level. The more details about the quality offered, the higher the level of functioning.

At a high level of awareness, clients are also able to delineate alternative qualities or subroles. For example, a client may speak of the temptations confronted by Pious—those times that she feels ambivalent toward her family and faith, as they stand in the way of realizing her sexual or aesthetic needs. Pious thus, assumes a greater moral complexity. At a lower level, clients are unaware of alternative qualities or subroles. At the lowest level, a role is a fixed, self-contained entity, with no possibility of movement beyond itself and no ambivalence as to its means of enactment. Thus Pious becomes, by definition and by deed, one who always chooses the righteous path and has no need to look back.

To assess the function of a role, the therapist either asks for it directly or in the form of this question: "How does the role serve the character?" In considering clients' responses, it may be useful to specify several levels of functioning. Level 1, the lowest level, represents either a denial or an inappropriate response (e.g., "The role of Pious doesn't serve any purpose at all," or "Pious looks out for herself."). Level 2 represents a response that focuses upon external objects or simple external causality (e.g., a client may state that the function of Pious is to dress in white, or that piety serves the character by leading her to do more good deeds).

Level 3 encompasses an unequivocal moral point of view, so that a role is seen as either good or bad, helpful or hurtful. A client, for example, may state that Pious is a moral character by nature and devotes her life, like Mother Teresa, to helping others in need. At Level 4, a client expresses a more open point of view, supported by empirical and/or intuitive evidence. For example, Pious may be seen as good because she has taken a stand against an oppressive government, or she has found the inner strength to speak out against the abuses of her father.

Finally, Level 5 represents the ability to attribute alternative meanings to a role and to live with role ambivalence. Thus, Pious may be seen as good not only because she has rebelled against an oppressive circumstance and devoted her professional life to helping victims of oppression, but also because she has allowed herself to play out her immoral side, at least in fantasy, and has learned to live with her own pulls toward oppression and expression. It would appear that clients functioning at Level 5 may hardly be in need of therapy. Yet some are so ambivalent and divergent in their thinking that there is little room for effective decision making or the expression of any feeling other than anxiety and depression. In such cases, therapy may well be indicated.

In order to better assess the balance of feeling and thinking, the therapist also looks at the style of role playing. At one extreme is the fully presentational style, marked by idiosyncratic, abstract movement and speech and by a detachment from the trappings of realism. In the extreme the client may even be unable or unwilling to express feeling. As noted earlier in this book, such a client is viewed by a drama therapist as overdistanced. At the other extreme is the fully representational style, too grounded in reality and marked by an abundance of affect, with scant room for reflection and critical thought. Such a client is underdistanced, too merged with the character on an emotional level.

In assessing the style of role playing, the therapist looks for the client's ability both to move through the spectrum of distance and to seek aesthetic distance (i.e., a balance of feeling and thought, of reality and abstraction). Both over- and underdistanced clients require the kind of treatment that will help them move toward balance as they play out their everyday roles.

Finally, the therapist asks the clients to talk about the connection between the fictional roles and their everyday lives. How is Pious, for example, played out on a daily basis? How do her qualities, functions, and style serve the person? Again, Levels 1–5 may aid in assessing this criterion. At Level 1, clients may see no connection between the fictional and the everyday. At Level 2, they may see that the Pious role makes them look better in the eyes of others. At Level 3, the clients may note that their piety allows them to feel moral and to push away all negative thoughts they have about themselves. At Level 4, the clients may see the Pious part as helping them get on with their work (e.g., as politically committed mental health professionals). And at Level 5, the clients may look more openly and critically not only at the ways the Pious role helps them function, but also at ways that it blocks them from acknowledging their need to be taken care of when they burn out. Furthermore, clients at this level may view their pious behavior in the context of their society and culture.

These five levels reflect a progression from a limited perspective to an ability to take on diverse points of view, similar to that offered in cognitive-developmental theories based on Piaget's research. Yet my intention is not simply cognitive and chronological, but rather holistic and psychological. Thus a numerical point on a continuum is insufficient in itself to diagnose a client according to the role method. All clients need to be encouraged to reveal a confluence of qualities, functions, and styles that well represents their ability to take on and play out roles, regardless of their ranking upon a 5-point scale. In taking these diagnostic suggestions a step further, the drama therapist needs to supplement the numerical assessment with a more qualitative narrative that offers a clinical impression of a client's well-being.

The point of the diagnosis is to assess how well clients are able to access their roles, play them out, and understand how they function in their lives on a number of different levels. For those who reveal difficulties in the ways and means of role playing, the dramatic role method may well be indicated as a treatment.

Despite the gains made in several dramatic instruments, a fully developed means of diagnosis based on the art form still eludes drama therapists. My remarks are intended to suggest further ways to diagnose clients, based on a conception of the human being as role recipient, role taker, and role player and based on the notion of healing dysfunctional roles and role systems through the dramatic role method.

EVALUATION

How does the therapist or researcher know whether the role method has been successful in treating such clients as Michael and Ann? Generally speaking, as any form of therapy begins to wind down, certain discernible shifts become apparent. In a behaviorally oriented therapy, a change in behavior will occur. In more psychodynamically oriented therapy, a client will have transformed unconscious issues into consciousness. Success in cognitive forms of therapy will lead to new ways of formulating and solving problems. In drama therapy practiced according to the role method, the shifts will occur within the role system and become apparent as revised roles are played out in everyday life. To evaluate those shifts, the therapist/researcher may modify the diagnostic criteria given above.

For one, therapy may be judged successful to the extent that clients are able to gain access to their role systems. That is, clients should be able to invoke those roles appropriate to a given circumstance and to play them out in a satisfying manner. For Michael, this might mean playing out intimate lover with Bill and adult son when in the presence of his mother and father. Following moments of regression, Michael should be able to reflect upon his role ambivalence and catch himself before a regressive role (e.g., the victim) usurps too much control over his role system.

An effective treatment should also account for the ability of clients to play out their roles in some depth, aware of the inherent ambiguities built into individual roles or caused by the collision of discrepant roles. At times, a superficial quality of role playing will prove quite appropriate—as, for example, when friends on the run exchange a quick greeting. Yet in constructing a deeper level of friendship, one will certainly need to develop more communicative and caring qualities.

Furthermore, successful clients should be able to play out a variety of roles, significantly expanding their role systems. For Ann, that might mean moving beyond rescuer, victim, and daughter in distress.

As the quantity of roles expands, Ann should be able to play out not only her rebellious roles, but also intimate and powerful ones (e.g., lover and friend, victor and independent woman).

In evaluating the expansion of clients' role systems, the therapist/researcher should keep in mind that the aim of treatment through the role method is not to extinguish dysfunctional roles, like so many undesirable behaviors. Dysfunctional roles remain part of the system as foils and balancers for the functional ones, just as, in the psychoanalytical system, id and superego remain even as the ego grows in its power to test reality appropriately. And the great psychological battles echo the mythological ones between demons and gods. Although the latter are victorious for a time, both demons and gods are eternally wedded to each other and will continue their dialectical battles in perpetuity.

When treatment has been successful, the dysfunctional roles undergo a transformation or revision. For Ann by the end of treatment, the rescuer part remained but was significantly less controlling. She noticed that it reared its head when, for example, she felt herself needing to rescue her lover. But she was usually able to see it in time, before it led her back into the kitchen with a needy and threatening father.

Thus, Ann and others like her may be judged successful to the extent that they are able to catch themselves before they fall headlong into old patterns. They need then to take a further step into enacting alternative ways of being. For Ann, the alternative to rescuing became the ability to allow herself to be held and nurtured when she felt needy. In allowing her lover and friends to provide that form of comfort, Ann began to move further away from the rescuer part of herself. A large measure of the effectiveness of the drama therapy will depend upon the ability of the client to take on and play out alternative role qualities, often embedded in subroles.

Furthermore, clients should be able to understand the ways that prominent roles function within their role systems. In understanding function, it is important that the client recognize not only the value of both positive and negative, original and revised roles; but also the more complicated ways that roles become entwined and often serve to pull a person in different directions. As we have seen above in the case of Hansel and Gretel, roles often intersect in ways that cause tension and ambivalence (e.g., Ann's rescuer–murderer configuration). In evaluating the effectiveness of the therapy, the therapist/researcher does not look for a resolution—that is, a victory of one role over the other—but rather a means of living in the ambivalence. In terms of role function, this means an understanding of the complementary purposes of two roles. For Ann, as we have seen, the murderer role worked hand in hand with that of the rescuer, serving as a reminder that in order to rescue herself she must kill off an image of a dysfunctional family.

In evaluating the treatment, the therapist or researcher should also look for the ability of the client to move through presentational and representational styles of role enactment, when appropriate. Well-functioning clients are those able to enact some roles with an abundance of feeling, others with an abundance of intellect, and still others alternating between the two. Too, clients should be free to abstract some roles some of the time, clowning, fooling around, and ridiculing—secure in the knowledge that when one takes on the head of an ass, like Bottom in *A Midsummer Night's Dream,* one is not necessarily destined to live the asinine life. On the other hand, the same clients should also feel free to play out their reality-based roles, again without fearing the permanent loss of the playful and critical parts of the psyche.

Thus successful treatment implies an ability to move through the spectrum of style and distance and, more often than not, to find a balance between feeling and thought, reality and illusion, so that roles can be taken on and off at will rather than at the bidding of some internalized god, parent, or victimizer. Clients who receive positive evaluations are able to invoke roles effectively, and then to play them and alternatives out in a style that well suits the role and the social circumstances. Furthermore, such clients would be able to attribute clear and meaningful functions to their roles. I would add that fully functional clients are also able to integrate their roles in such a way that a fluid system is created. By "fluid," I mean a system in which one role can move easily within the compass of another when needed (e.g., like the rescuer and murderer roles of Ann, and the heartless woman and helpless child roles of Julia). Although these roles are not exactly opposites, they do create tension when combined. Within that tension lies a powerful healing potential. If the roles are fluid, they can combine to help an individual work through a difficult problem.

Ultimately, the value of the role method lies in its view of individuals as capable of solving their own problems through a reconfiguration of their roles. The drama therapist serves as a guide throughout the process. At the conclusion of successful therapy, those roles that have been rigid are more fluid; those lying dormant are more accessible; those tyrannizing the system are less controlling. In effective drama therapy, a client reaches a balance or integration of roles, which paradoxically shifts when the person seeks out or is confronted with new challenges. The role system is powered by role ambivalence, a state of affairs that sparks learning, creativity, and healing.

In evaluation, the therapist or researcher most highly values a person who is not simply balanced, but capable of coping with imbalance—the chaos of contradictory qualities and styles, of hard choices presented by two conflicting but equally compelling points of view. Such a person is recognized by an ability to live in the ambivalence of being; to be one and many, real and abstract, feelingful thinker and reflective actor; to be *and* not to be at the same time. As a social role model, this is the person best equipped to pass on to others a wisdom born of paradox and ambivalence. Such a person is hard to see from the outside.

In conceptualizing such a person from the inside, I have been pointing to a model of an interactive role system. Such a system develops by virtue of genetic, social, and behavioral factors whereby roles are given, taken, and played out. The dramatic role model consists of role types that are differentiated according to specific qualities, functions, and styles of enactment. As we have seen, the dramatic role model is useful in treatment through drama therapy as it takes the shape of the dramatic role method. In the previous several chapters, two case studies involving such treatment have been presented. Suggestions have been offered as to means of diagnosing and evaluating clients in treatment.

In the following chapters, I propose to extend the dramatic role model further by looking at potential ways that role types can be organized, and thus attempting to reveal the contents of the role system. This exploration is important, in that it can shed further light on clinical treatment through the role method as clients attempt to understand and reconfigure their role systems. Such an approach may further pave the way for a more comprehensive theory of role by establishing the critical links among drama, therapy, and everyday life.

The next chapter focuses upon the organization of roles taken on and played out in everyday life. Following that, I move back to the primary source of role, that of theatre, and attempt to delineate many of the most often repeated role types in the form of a taxonomy. Roles from everyday life and theatre are chosen on the basis of the extent to which they recapitulate certain basic archetypal forms.

CHAPTER SEVEN

Role in Everyday Life

ROLE TYPE AND ARCHETYPE

The question of typing in everyday life and theatre is a thorny one, in that complexity of character tends to be highly valued in both areas. The concept of "stereotype" is itself a pejorative one; it connotes a reducing, diminishing, or. belittling of a person. Yet a reduction of the complexity of the human personality into discrete, comprehensible forms is the work of artists and healers alike, who attempt to make sense of the whole by isolating and focusing on selected parts. Stereotyping certainly does reduce the person through oversimplification and cliché. But that is not the aim of psychological typologists such C. G. Jung (1921/1971), who search for underlying personality structures; or literary typologists such as Vladimir Propp (1968), who search for underlying narrative structures; or biological typologists such as Stephen Jay Gould (1989), who search for new ways to taxonomize ancient forms of life, allowing us to see the full spectrum of evolution more clearly. Typing at its best is a method of selection through framing certain phenomena, based upon specified criteria.

Jung was one of the early psychological typologists, categorizing human beings in terms of four functions (sensation, thinking, feeling, and intuition) and two general attitudes (introversion and extroversion). According to Jung (1921/1971), there are eight potential psychological types: the introverted sensation type, the extroverted sensation type, and the introverted and extroverted thinking, feeling, and intuitive types. Although Jung's typology proved useful in conceptualizing personality types, his descriptions were sometimes confused and contradictory. Jung's reputation as a typologist is more firm-ly based upon his more poetic conception of "archetype." In an ex-haustive cross-cultural analysis of the mythic, symbolic, and collective nature of the human personality, Jung (1964) demonstrated how in-dividuals tend to take on and play out in their everyday lives the universal themes and archetypal roles subsisting in history, literature, art, religion, and mythology. These dramatic tendencies appear to be inherited, deposited within the collective unconscious of each hu-man being.

Many Jungians have taken their investigations to arcane places (as did Jung himself), examining UFOs, alchemy, astrology, and eso-teric mystical texts. Although some of this research appears frivolous, the Jungian canon is rich in metaphor and germane to a central theme of this book: namely, that there are repeated types and forms that subsist in the body, mind, and spirit of human beings. These forms can be named and traced to specific sources. Jung called them "arche-types", and found their sources in the myths and symbols of diverse cultures. Through an analysis of the archetypes and integration of the conscious mind with the unconscious archetypal material, Jung believed that an individual should be able to move toward healthy psychological functioning—a state that he called "individ-uation."

Throughout this book, the theatrical term "role type" is in many ways equivalent to the psychological term "archetype." Like Jung, I attempt to demonstrate how universal forms repeat themselves both in clinical situations and in everyday life. Furthermore, like Jung, I argue that the archetypal roles need to be identified and integrated within one's personality structure or role system in order to develop healthy psychological functioning.

I depart from the Jungians in several ways. For one, the Jungian archetypal system tends to be a catch-all for many kinds of esoteric thinkers and practitioners, leading to a discipline with such wide parameters that the center does not often hold. In its quest for cross-cultural and transpersonal knowledge, the field of archetypal psychol-ogy tends to become too enigmatic, at once overly intellectual and overtly mystical. In some instances, the search for cross-cultural arche-types translates poorly and vaguely into clinical practice.

In addition, the Jungian system of healing is an analytical one. As such, the analysts hold a considerable degree of power, sometimes taking on the role of seer or oracle. The patients' role as healer of their own problems can thus become diminished. Many Jungian analysts, like their mentor, use expressive means of healing, through a process that Jung called "active imagination." For others, however, the creative process is minimally integrated into the mainstream of treatment; when it is, it tends to be a means toward the analytical end.

This chapter classifies and describes a number of roles readily available in everyday life. The following chapters provide a more complete archetypal system of roles related to those specified in everyday life, yet based solidly in theatre and expressed in the form of a taxonomy. Like Jung, I have a need to specify many of the role types that inform our lives and that, when imbalanced, block the development of an integrated personality. It is not my intention to suggest that roles exist in isolation. Although they are conceptualized as such, it is with the understanding that in reality, roles interact and intersect in complex ways. Some, like Jungian archetypes, coexist in "fearful symmetry" suggested by Blake in "The Tyger" (1794/1960)—a paradoxical balance of potentially explosive qualities.

Roles in everyday life can be organized within six broad categories: somatic, cognitive, affective, social/cultural, spiritual, and aesthetic. These categories are not arbitrary, but respond to the central concerns of those physicians, philosophers, psychologists, sociologists, anthropologists, theologians, and artists who continue to probe the body, mind, feelings, soul and habitat of humankind. Throughout this discussion, everyday roles are specified according to type, quality, and function, when relevant. This chapter also addresses the question of the origins of many of the roles presented.

SOMATIC ROLES

Survival Roles

Somatic roles, primarily inherited and genetically based, pertain to the body—as it functions, as it develops, and as it appears. The first class encompasses those roles necessary for one's survival. Examples include the roles of breather, sucker, eater, expeller, sleeper, mover, and interactor. The role of procreator also falls into this category.

Survival roles undergo many changes as they are played throughout a person's life. Thus, the quality and often the function of the roles will change from childhood to old age, even though the nature of the roles remains constant. As an example, people will play out the role of eater throughout their lives as a way of nourishing themselves. Yet the eater as child may little resemble the eater as adolescent, adult, or elder. The young child may resist food, play with food, or gulp it down in order to move on to more exciting or less demanding tasks. The adolescent may begin to associate food with physical appearance and use it as a means toward shaping a more culturally desirable persona. The adult may learn to take sensual pleasure in food and expend much energy in its creation, consumption, and critique. The elder, on the other hand, may view food as simply a necessity and take scant delight in its preparation. Furthermore, changes in economic circumstances, environment (e.g., moving from a home to an institution) and inner psychological state (e.g., moving from a point of emotional balance to one of depression) will signal for many a change in their conception and enactment of the eater role.

Age and Developmental Stage

A second classification of somatic roles has to do with age and developmental stage. Age roles include the child, the adolescent, the adult, and the elder. Each age role or developmental stage is based upon a range of ages. Childhood extends until puberty (roughly 12 years of age), followed by adolescence, which stretches until the end of the teens. The adult role extends until retirement age or senior citizen status (approximately 65 years of age), followed by the elder years, which Erikson (1963) has characterized as those embodying the struggle between despair and wisdom.

Each chronological, developmental stage is not only biologically determined, but also psychologically based. A 7-year-old may function at the cognitive level of an average 14-year-old; an adolescent may behave as a child. Role reversals are common: For example, frail elderly people may regress to the dependent status of children because of illness and isolation, and children may be thrust prematurely into adult roles because of such circumstances as poverty, divorce, and death. In these and similar examples, the elder as child or child as adult has, in part, chosen the role reversal. That choice, however, is mitigated by given physiological, psychological, or cultural circumstances. For example, the patient with severe Alzheimer's disease has a limited ability to play out appropriate adult roles. The young girl whose parents have died in a terrorist bombing apparently has more choice. She may choose, among other options, to take on an adult role and play mother to her brother, or to stay within the parameters of the child role and search out alternative parents.

A curious cultural phenomenon has developed among some inner-city adolescents in the United States, who have chosen to take on the role of infant (as demonstrated by sucking on baby bottles, pacifiers, and thumbs in private and public). Given a rising number of murders and suicides among this group,* as well as incidents of

*According to FBI statistics (1991), the arrest rate for people under 18 increased 60% between 1981 and 1990. And according to the National Institute of Mental Health (1989), the rate of suicide among adolescents increased 92% from 1970 to 1989.

12- and 13-year-olds attending school with handguns and automatic weapons, perhaps this phenomenon is not so curious. If adolescents growing up in abject poverty and psychologically threatening environments are forced to deny their youth, they may well take comfort in regressing to a more primitive stage of greater psychological security. If it is true that some of these same individuals have also been denied a psychologically healthy childhood within an intact family, the regression is that much more poignant. For adolescents who have experienced more than their share of adult violence and neglect, the need for an emotional pacifier contained within the role of the infant is great.

Gender and Sex Roles

Gender and sexuality represent a third classification of somatic roles. Like other somatic role classes, gender is determined by nature but seems influenced by nurture. Influences are broad. One source is the family as a repository of masculine and feminine role models to be taken on by the child and subsequently played out. Another source is the culture, which offers images of masculinity and femininity and establishes norms in which to play out such views. And a third source consists of psychological factors, which provide an internal sense of identity as male and/or female. Given the incorporation of conventional expectations from family and culture, one tends to view oneself in a conventional way as to gender.

However, gender roles do not necessarily conform to the male and female stereotypes prevalent in a culture. As cultures become more heterogeneous and permissive, more choices are available as to how and when one will play out one's feminine or masculine roles. With the advent of feminism and the subsequent men's movement, people take on new role models and explore new ways to play out their given gender roles. And given a powerful psychological model of integration, like that proposed by Jung (1964), men and women have begun to search within their psyches for a sexual counterpart. According to Jung, the male archetype, or animus, needs to be integrated by women, just as the female archetype, or anima, needs to be integrated by men to achieve a healthy sexual balance.

Biology, culture, and psychology sometimes collude in obfuscating the clear lines between masculine and feminine. This happens when one is born as a biological man, for example, and is reinforced to choose masculine pursuits, yet feels like a woman. In such unusual cases, as well as more ordinary ones of confused gender identity, a clue to understanding the genesis of gender roles may be found in the role models that have been internalized. If these can be known, we may move a step closer to understanding the quality and form of a person's role playing.

Concurrent with the struggle to discover a balanced sense of masculinity and femininity is the struggle to take on and play out a satisfactory sexual identity as gay, heterosexual, bisexual, asexual, or some combination. Some, out of religious convictions, choose to remain celibate. Others, fearing death or illness through AIDS or other sexually transmitted diseases, may also choose to abstain. And in the image fostered by a culture reacting intensely against a former period of sexual permissiveness, still others may choose to remain asexual either as a moral statement or as a hip, cultural one. Yet it is not clear whether one chooses one's sexual orientation.

Nature still tends to be the most compelling determinant of one's sexuality (see, e.g., Marmor, 1980, and Tripp, 1987). Nurture's contribution, as seen above, consists of a confluence of family, culture, and psychology (see Byne, 1988a, 1988b). The pool of social role models available in a given environment supports one's search for an appropriate sexual role.

Appearance Roles

A fourth somatic classification concerns roles related to appearance. The two extreme role types found time and again in myth and fairy tale are those of beauty and the beast. In the fairy tale of the same name, the character Beauty is not only lovely to look at, but also highly moral, an innocent as well as a beauty. The role type of beauty pertains primarily to physical qualities. It becomes more complex when moral qualities are introduced in terms of beauty as innocent versus beauty as seductive.

The beast as role type is the opposite of beauty—ugly, unpleasing in face and shape, sometimes deformed. On a moral level, the beast may embody a demonic quality or a hidden goodness; for example, the Beast of the fairy tale is transformed to a prince when loved by Beauty. There are many examples of deformed characters in fiction whose external ugliness masks an innocence or inner beauty (e.g., the monster in Mary Shelley's [1818/1983] *Frankenstein* and the title character in the film *Edward Scissorhands*, a monster-like boy with hands made of razor-sharp scissors and a heart of gold).

A third appearance role is that of the average one. This type is characterized by plain looks and average stature. Again, taking on and playing out the role of the average one constitute more than a simple statement of appearance. To be average implies an acceptance of limitations. The possibility of a glamorous and powerful life remains at the level of fantasy. In some cases, the role of the average one implies an existential state of alienation, a sense of being lost in the universe. Others, who conceive of themselves as less than average (e.g., abnormal, stigmatized, or disabled in some essential way), may strive toward the average role as a way to feel more acceptable and connected to the mainstream.

Looks are inherited. Yet the mirror that offers the final judgment as to appearance reflects changing fashions and changing self-images. These changes occur as people interact with others and take on their perspectives. For instance, if someone else sees me as beautiful, I see myself the same way; beauty is thus situated in the eyes of both beholder and beheld. In a like manner, the roles of beast and average one are taken on from others. For people to live truly functional lives in terms of appearance means for them to interact effectively with their beholders, allowing their beautiful, beastly, and ordinary qualities to take shape in the roles they play.

Health Roles

Health is a fifth general classification within the somatic domain. The types of roles to be found in this category include the physically fit person, as well as both the mentally ill and the physically disabled.

Many health roles develop some time after birth, even though many specific illnesses or tendencies toward sickness–wellness are inherited. When health roles become more psychosomatically based, the individual may well be choosing a particular dysfunctional role for a particular purpose, which many times remains unconscious. An example is that of a person who suffers from migraine headaches, which, although physiologically based, can be triggered by acute stress and unconsciously chosen as a means of avoidance. The psychosomatic role, then, is a transitional one that falls somewhere in between physical and emotional illness.

Another role type, that of the hypochondriac, is characterized by a pretense of being sick. Many actually believe their own pretense and see themselves as ill. Such people are similar to the boy who cries wolf, in that they feign illness in order to protect themselves from imagined fears. Usually foolish in appearance, hypochondriacs manage to draw an inordinate amount of attention to themselves.

COGNITIVE ROLES

Cognitive roles concern one's way of thinking through and solving problems. Lower-level cognitive tasks, such as the recall of factual information, imply a different quality of role playing than higher-level tasks, such as synthesis and evaluation (see Bloom, David, & Masia, 1956). Many attempts at describing and categorizing cognitive processes tend to be hierarchical, moving from less to more knowledge or from lower- to higher-level cognitive skills.

In their *Taxonomy of Educational Objectives* for the cognitive domain, Bloom et al. (1956) present a well-reasoned hierarchy proceeding from knowledge to comprehension, application, analysis, synthesis, and evaluation. It may well be that each cognitive objective implies a corresponding cognitive role: the one who (like the accountant Sam, described in Chapter Two) collects facts; the one who makes sense of the facts from an empirical point of view; the one who applies an understanding of the facts to other information; the analytical person, who is able to interpret the facts according to certain prescribed criteria; the synthesizer, who is able to construct new ideas based upon an integration of old ones; and the evaluator, who is able to measure or judge the value of ideas.

An old Arabic maxim reduces cognitive roles to four—the fool, the simple one, the sleeper, and the wise one (see Scheff, 1979, p. 166):

He who knows not and knows not that he knows not, he is a fool. Shun him.
He who knows not and knows that he knows not, he is simple. Teach him.
He who knows and knows not that he knows, he is asleep. Awake him.
He who knows and knows that he knows, he is wise. Follow him.

Although this hierarchy expresses a more dramatic and poetic sense of role, it also applies to cognitive roles appearing in everyday life. For example, we all play the fool at times in our lives. As given in the maxim, however, this type is in some ways a misnomer, as classical fools often mask superior intelligence and cunning in a suit of motley and a diminished status. Even such modern popular fools as Charlie Chaplin and Woody Allen work as much through irony and wit as through slapstick.

The lowest-order cognitive role for our purposes is the simpleton rather than the fool—more Laurel than Hardy, more Three Stooges than the Marx Brothers. These are character types who remain unaware of their ignorance. We laugh at them because they restimulate our own ignorance and allow us to discharge our embarrassment. The highest-order role, that of the knowingly wise person, remains basically the same as given in the maxim above. Many an intellectual aspires to this role, but most fall short, mired in ambivalence, criticism, and pedantry.

In between the simpleton and the wise person lie other cognitive roles. The sleeper may be equivalent to the humble or self-deprecating intellectual, who toils away un-self-consciously, with little concern or awareness of the value of his discoveries. Other examples of cognitive roles include the ambivalent one, he who knows this and knows that, but doesn't know whether this or that is a more significant choice; the lost one, he who once knew but now does not even know that he knew; and the critic and the pedant, they who think they know and think they know that they know.

Many cognitive models, whether scientifically or poetically based, point to a way of viewing cognitive roles as developmental and hierarchical. Piaget (Piaget & Inhelder, 1969) and such prominent disciples as Kohlberg and Lickona (1986) in moral development and Selman et al. (1982) in social-cognitive development (see Chapter Two) offer a compelling body of research attesting to the development of thought according to certain prescribed stages. By implication, cognitive roles, then, are acquired in an invariable sequence as the individual moves from a singular, egocentric perspective to a multiple, decentered one. Yet this linear approach should not be seen as the only way that cognitive roles come into being.

A more dialectical model may also be useful in conceptualizing cognitive roles. The character Hamlet, for example, though chronologically an adolescent or young adult, assumes a variety of cognitive roles (some of which are contradictory) within a short space of time. He is both simpleton and wise man, fool and sleeper. He appears at times to be both knowledgeable and ignorant of the facts of the political and psychological landscapes of Denmark. He is both able and unable to apply his knowledge toward a resolution of his existential dilemma. He is, furthermore, both analytical and irrational—on the one hand, correctly interpreting the events that have led to the rotten state of Danish affairs; and on the other, overwhelmed by his ambivalences and thus unable to act. Hamlet's final role, that of the vengeful man of action, is effective to the extent that it decimates the passivity of his analytical role, which keeps him mired in doubt, indecision, and rationalization throughout most of the play.

Shakespeare's play offers a complex portrait of one who lives in many ways in his mind, and develops in a number of directions at once, according to his psychology rather than an imposed chronology. As in Hamlet's case, the cognitive roles we inherit or take on or play out in the social world may develop circuitously, through our interactions with the shifting and often contradictory pulls of that world.

AFFECTIVE ROLES

Affective roles concern values and feelings. On the one hand, they represent moral values of the kind that appear in fables, folk tales, and religious teachings. They can be found in such diverse sources as the didactic German children's stories about Messy Peter, who is severely punished every time he disobeys his mother, and the dialectical *Songs of Innocence and of Experience* by the Romantic poet and artist, William Blake.

Affective roles also represent feeling states—at one extreme, the impulsive extrovert, overwhelmed by feeling; at the other, the compulsive introvert, fearful of emotional expression.

Moral Roles

The basic moral values displayed through affective roles are those representing the interplay of good and evil, innocence and experience. Often these roles are presented as conflicting with one another: the virgin and the whore, the martyr and the opportunist, and the helper and the deceiver, for example.

Young children may invent a bad or naughty role to contain their unacceptable actions and feelings. Thus, when Susan has dropped her plate on the floor, scattering the food and breaking the glass, she may attribute the action to "Doreen," a demonic role of her invention.

Adolescence becomes a stage upon which endless moral struggles are played out. Those roles that have been taken on in childhood are significantly expanded or locked in. A 13-year-old victim of early sexual abuse may seek out role models in others who have been abused, or, identifying with the aggressor, may search for others to victimize. A second adolescent victim may take on the martyr role, playing out in a Christ-like fashion the part of the suffering servant. This role may well serve the needs of a dysfunctional family that unconsciously designates one member to shoulder its pathologies. The chosen one, as martyr, will bear the burdens silently and stoically, thus protecting the others from acknowledging their complicity in the cycle of abuse and denial. A third abused adolescent may search for more positive role models—those of helpers, healers, or teachers, who provide an alternative approach to repeating the cycle of pain.

The seeds of morality are planted in childhood and blossom in adolescence in the form of moralists and immoralists, victims and victimizers, magnanimous ones and bigots. These roles exist internally as they are taken on from the social world represented by peers, parents, and other authority figures. Once the moral roles have established firm root systems, the adult moral figure appears. That is not to say that adults are fixed in their moral roles, but that for the most part they tend to resist changing their moral structures. The shift of a moral role is somewhat like a religious conversion. When it does appear, it requires deep personal conviction and a willingness to confront the inherent ambivalences.

At the end of the 20th century, which has been marked too often by systematic attempts at enslavement and genocide, the sense of moral role playing seems based more often than not on denial of responsibility by those who might speak out and act. In denial, the moral role does not disappear; instead, it turns inward, leading to a sense of oneself as good or bad, innocent or responsible, or somewhere in between. And even in the overt expression of one's morality, one does not necessarily resolve the inner moral struggles that need to be expressed repeatedly in order to assert one's moral position in the world. The richest moral role models are those who can act in the world morally and also acknowledge their ongoing inner struggles between the forces of righteousness and immorality.

Feeling States

The sociologist Scheff (1979) specifies three feeling states: underdistance, overdistance, and aesthetic distance. Each can be translated into a role that well embodies the degree of affect.

The first feeling state, that of underdistance, is exemplified by the manic, impulsive one who is too much out of control, flooded with feeling, tending to identify too powerfully with a single role and to merge too fully with other people. Underdistancing can be observed in the behavior of a hotheaded coach, such as the late Billy Martin, who was known to kick sand in the face of an occasional despised umpire. Examples of underdistanced affective roles include the hothead, the angry young man/woman, and the ecstatic or possessed one under the spell of an intoxicant. In the case of Michael, we have seen examples of underdistanced behavior as he invoked the Black Rage. Michael as angry young man is well exemplified in his story "The Boy Who Learned to Burn" (see Chapter Four).

The role of the overdistanced one is the opposite: Too much control is at work with too little feeling, causing a wide separation between actor and role, individual and other. An extreme example is the zombie, one who plays at being dead or deadened. The highly stylized zombies in horror movies mirror actual roles played by those who deny their feelings at all costs. Michael also took on some overdistanced roles, such as that of the blind, beaten-down, abused young girl, Patty.

The distancing model from which these roles are derived is conceptualized as a continuum (Scheff, 1979; Landy, 1983) where the midpoint is aesthetic distance, a balance of affect and cognition. Aesthetic distance is an ideal state in which one is able to think feelingly and feel without the fear of being overwhelmed with passion. Csikszent-mihalyi (1990) has conceptualized this state as "flow," a point of spontaneity that marks effective experiences in problem solving, creativity, and human relations. When in "flow" or at aesthetic distance, an individual is able to be playful, responding spontaneously to new experience and revisiting old experience as if for the first time. Aesthetic distance is the optimal feeling state that applies to the creative process, as experienced in the arts and sciences, in the home, in the workplace, or on the playground.

In assuming feeling states, one generally exhibits a degree of aesthetic distance, which may vary greatly with changing circumstances. It is very difficult to predict how individuals will play out affective roles. Factors to consider include family role models, cultural expectations as to acceptable expression of emotion, psychological predisposition, and environmental circumstances. In extreme external circumstances (e.g., war), one who appears meek but has great inner resources might perform heroic acts. In more ordinary circumstances, a person who has internalized a strong sense of shame may impose that trait on an otherwise neutral situation, such as a minor rebuff from a supervisor at work.

The roles related to feeling states tend to be fluid as one moves throughout the spectrum of distance. In extreme cases of over- and underdistance, a form of therapy is indicated that can help restore balance and flow.

SOCIAL/CULTURAL ROLES

Social and cultural roles reflect ways that people organize themselves in groups of families, communities, societies, and states. Cultural roles further address issues of ethnicity, as well as morality, religion, age, gender, sexuality, and disability. We speak frequently of the youth culture, the gay culture, the deaf culture, the Jewish culture, or the feminist culture, for example.

Society and culture, taken together, are powerful determinants of how, when, and why we take on and play out our roles. Those who identified with the youth culture of the late 1960s and early 1970s not only took on the required appearance, values, and beliefs, but also a sense of how to play out their roles. Most also had a sense of why the youth role was important—as a statement of rebellion, liberation, and joy, similar to that experienced by many people living through a political revolution. The role of hippie or the more politicized yippie was taken on consciously. Moreover, like many religious or political movements, the youth movement was tied in with certain significant historical event (e.g., the bombing of Cambodia and the various peace marches on Washington during the Vietnam war, the Chicago riots and the subsequent trial of the Chicago Seven following the 1968 Democratic convention, and the galvanizing Woodstock festival). The youth role models of the day—including Bob Dylan and Joan Baez, the Rolling Stones and the Doors, Jimi Hendrix and Janis Joplin, Abbie Hoffman and Angela Davis—provided the prototypes for a youth culture of protest, drugs, sex, and rock and roll. Large social movements, like those occurring within the women's, youth, and black communities in the late 1960s throughout much of the Western world, tend to shape roles, even as those who are already en-roled shape the movements. The society and culture offer a pool of roles to be taken on. The individual, in taking on and playing out certain key roles at certain key historical times, becomes a role model for others seeking to participate in a significant cultural or historical event.

It could be argued that many cultural roles are primary, in that they are given at birth. Although they are not essential for biological survival, they are crucial in providing a clear sense of identity. One example is that of ethnicity. Ethnic roles are given to the extent that one is born, for example, Chicano/Chicana, African-American, Jewish, Arab, or Hopi. Yet there is great variety within ethnic groups as individuals choose which ethnic qualities they will take on and play out. The less traditional a culture, the more choice one will have.

Furthermore, some people will identify with the subcultural roles of those belonging to a different ethnic group. Within a prison environment, for example, many whites of various ethnic backgrounds will take on the speech and gesture of their black or Hispanic peers, whom they may view as the most powerful individuals on the block. Within such a closed society, moreover, a tendency toward conforming to a single tough, invulnerable role will pervade inmates and staff alike. In many ways, those who reject the prototypical tough inmate role take a great risk. Such a role becomes primary to the extent that it is essential for survival within the institution. Most institutions offer their own sets of cultural roles and demand a prescribed way of implementation: in the prison culture, the inmate role; in the military culture, the soldier role; in the corporate culture, the business role.

Social roles are perhaps the most obvious forms of role playing in everyday life. Social psychologists tend to view such roles deterministically; that is, they believe that role determines behavior and is itself determined by one's social environment. In much of the social-psychological literature (see, e.g., Cooley, 1922; Linton, 1936; Goffman, 1959), role is depicted as a collection of rights and duties associated with one's social status.

Family Roles

Some family roles are given—daughter and son, sister and brother, and a variety of blood relatives. The roles of wife and husband, father and mother, or less conventional forms of marriage and procreation are taken on. Whether family roles are given or chosen, the ways they are internalized and played out vary considerably.

When one examines roles within any given family, some form of hierarchy is generally apparent in terms of power, control, and decision making. Although this structure changes along with external circumstances (such as the loss of a job or a death in the family) or internal circumstances (such as a change of consciousness stemming from a political, spiritual, or therapeutic experience), the qualities of each family role maintain a strong hold on each family member. Family role definitions are reinforced in endless ways within a given culture. So too are they archetypally determined, reappearing cross-culturally in the forms of myth and icon that bombard one's everyday existence. A traditional family hierarchy, based in myth and culture, will seem familiar to those raised with the sensibility embedded in television situation comedies, from *Father Knows Best* to *The Cosby Show.*

The father/husband can be seen as the highest-status family role. The father is powerful, rational, and in control. He makes the most important decisions in the family and is its primary economic supporter. He embodies the imagery of God the Father, patriarch, king, priest, merchant and entrepreneur, provider and protector, dictator and president, captain of the ship, and master (though often absent) of the house. The status of father carries the rights of fealty, respect, and domestic tranquility. His duties include not only providing for and protecting his family, but also passing on his legacy to his children—teaching his son, especially, how to be a father.

The conventional role of the mother/wife can be seen as secondary to that of the father/husband; she is number two in the chain of command. Her power and control lie in her ability to nurture and take care of the father and children. She is more a person of affect, providing a moral base for the family and teaching the lessons of the heart. In visual and verbal imagery, she is depicted as the earth mother, queen, matriarch, goddess, priestess, nurturer, mistress of the house, and keeper of the hearth, omnipresent and reliable. She too may play a vocational role, but it is subordinate in status to that of the husband. The rights given to the mother are protection, security, and loyalty. Her duty is the maintenance of the emotional and domestic well-being of the family.

The role of the son, who is number three in status, is to perpetuate the image of the father, slowly internalizing his role and assuming his duties and responsibilities. The first-born son, the prince, thus becomes a king-in-training. He is expected to play masculine games, study masculine subjects, and master masculine skills. It is his right to inherit the legacy of his father, as well as to internalize the values of his mother.

The daughter role is conventionally the lowest in status. Her duties are to help her mother, all the while internalizing the mother role, and to aid her father in perpetuating his power. She receives a dowry without the power associated with a son's inheritance. When there are no sons, the daughter role is elevated in status: She will inherit real property, but only after proving her worthiness through emotional means. Like Lear's daughters, she must first convince her father of her love for him. Her rights, therefore, are minimal, associated with flattery, love, and loyalty.

Another historically significant family role is that of the elder or grandparent. The traditional duties of elders are to pass on their wisdom to the parents concerning child-rearing practices, and to pass on a kind of moral code to the children.

The interaction patterns among these traditionally drawn roles are quite complex. Specific cultures establish certain principles and taboos to help maintain the role definitions. Freud used the dramatic character Oedipus to highlight the primary Western family taboo against incest. He posited that psychological development recapitulates the ancient dramas of Oedipus and the House of Atreus, wherein sons harbored incestuous feelings toward mothers and homicidal feelings toward fathers. In one version, detailed in *Totem and Taboo* (1913/1960), Freud spoke of the primal horde or ancient tribe, presided over by a jealous patriarch who controlled the women and banished the sons once they reached sexual maturity. Collectively, the sons rose up against the father, murdered him, and ritually consumed his body as a way of taking on his power and status. Yet, in their ambivalent feelings toward the loved and despised father, the sons experienced guilt. To assuage their guilt, they proclaimed the act of parricide forbidden and denied themselves the women once belonging to the father. This, according to Freud, marked the beginning of civilization and morality, with clear prohibitions against role confusion and clear definitions of conventional ways of playing out family roles.

Although Freud was much less precise and poetic regarding the "Electra complex," he presumed that the daughter at an early stage of psychosexual development similarly fosters an unconscious desire for the father and anger toward the mother for her possession of such a valued object.

The picture of family roles painted above is still a reality for many who model and take on family roles. Yet for many who are more directly affected by contemporary cultural realities, family roles have been significantly revised and transformed. Because of divorces and subsequent second and third marriages, husbands and wives may live with the children of a spouse, some of whom may be old enough to be their siblings or at least their peers. In fact, according to the 1990 statistics from the U.S. Bureau of the Census, 21% of American households with children had at least one stepchild living with the family. For African-American households alone, that statistic rose to 33%.

Mothers have assumed the primary caretaker and breadwinner roles in many households. According to the U.S. Bureau of Census, the distribution of families with children in 1990 showed that 19% of white families were headed by single mothers. The statistics jumped significantly in regard to Hispanic and African-American families: 29% of Hispanic families and 33% of African-American families were led by single mothers. As the only adult figures within families devoid of adult males, single mothers assume all conventional qualities of both father and mother. Single fathers, who comprised 4% of the population in all three ethnic groups, likewise assume the dual roles of mother and father.

Some women have chosen to have children alone, without the financial help or presence of a father. With the advent of the feminist movement, the roles of women have been transformed significantly, leading to a reconceptualization of the family roles of wife and mother.

Children, too, are subject to the changing values of their parents, who may substitute the friend role for the parent role or disavow the parent role altogether, playing child to their own children. Such children have been nudged into abandoning a conventional understanding of their family roles. When children are deprived of their childhood—that is, of their rights to play and be cared for by responsible adults—there may be devastating emotional consequences in adulthood. This cultural phenomenon has been well documented by Alice Miller (see *The Drama of the Gifted Child,* 1981; *For Your Own Good,* 1983; and *Thou Shalt Not Be Aware: Society's Betrayal of the Child,* 1986).

Yet even during a time of ambivalence and change, the conventional role definitions do not go away. Society has too much at stake in preserving them. The electronic and print media still advertise a conventional family system. And most parents—whether single or married, whether straight or gay, and regardless of psychopolitical orientations—still carry within them the seeds of both stereotype and archetype, of social cliché and cultural building block.

Political and Legal Roles

A second class of social roles concerns political philosophy and status. Within this class, one type of role concerns the government of the community. At the top is one who serves in a leadership role (e.g., chief, elder, king, queen, president, or governor), whether appointed or elected or instated by force. Under the leader are various advisors, ministers, law enforcers, soldiers, legal officials, and bureaucrats of all kinds.

In playing out the variety of governmental roles, one tends to express oneself through a particular political philosophy, whether explicit or implicit. Each philosophy represents another political role, expressed through the spectrum of reactionary, conservative, liberal, pacifist, and revolutionary. Both the right and left ends of the spectrum imply ways of organizing, analyzing, and evaluating knowledge.

Related to political roles are those concerning the legal system, which in repressive societies is very much in the service of the state. Legal roles pertain to the interpretation of laws that govern the state, and the prosecution and defense of those accused of violating such laws. Within the legal system, people assume such roles as lawyer and prosecutor, defendant and witness, judge and jury. The role of jury takes on a special meaning within a democratic society, in that it is comprised of peers rather than experts. The jury becomes a populist tribunal, a voice of the people, a kind of Greek chorus that offers a consensual, "average" point of view.

Socioeconomic Roles

The spectrum of socioeconomic roles includes four classes: the lower class, the domain of the homeless person, welfare recipient, beggar, and peasant; the working class, represented by the blue-collar worker; the middle class, home of the skilled worker, businessperson, health care worker, legal official, educator and other professionals; and the upper class, station of the aristocrat and socialite, as well as the highly successful professional or entrepreneur.* One's socioeconomic status is very much interwoven with the political realities of

a community or culture. Many traditional Third World societies perpetuate a rigid class or caste system, despite developing economic,
political, and technological sophistication.

It would appear that socioeconomic roles are given and thus
primary, especially in traditional cultures where one is born poor, dies
poor, and leaves a legacy of the same to one's children. Yet class and
caste systems have evolved to the point at which birth is only one
factor determining role status. Since the flowering of the middle class
during the Industrial Revolution, one has been able to take on a
higher-status role by means of opportunity, initiative, and sometimes
exploitation. Thus workers and merchants, by virtue of their socioeconomic mobility, have transformed primary social roles into secondary ones.

Despite the different origins of class roles, each presents certain
discernible qualities. For example, in assuming their rights and
privileges, upper-class people consume and enjoy many of life's
material luxuries. They also demonstrate their power by influencing
government through financing political campaigns or accepting
nominations or appointments for high office. The targets of political and religious revolutionaries for centuries, they have neverthe-
less managed to survive relatively intact as a class, remaining a prime
focus of media attention from *People* magazine to the television pro-
gram *Lifestyles of the Rich and Famous.*

The middle-class role has been much satirized in its incarnation
as the bourgeoisie. Since its early development in the Renaissance,
the middle class has been portrayed as lacking in culture and sensibility. In its aspiration for the respectable and comfortable life, it has
taken on a value system best characterized as conservative in politics, philistine in culture, and materialist in commerce.

The working class comprises the target group of Marxist ideology. The working-class role is not necessarily motivated by acquiring

---

*Eric Miller—publisher of *Research Alert*, a publication that analyzes over a thousand
research reports on consumer trends each year—has informed me (personal communication, 1992) that although the Bureau of the Census will not provide a definition
for "middle class," he reads the Bureau's statistics as implying a steady shrinkage of that
group since 1967. This is verified by the rise in numbers of affluent households ($50,000+
a year in inflation-adjusted 1990 constant-dollar income since 1967) from 18.7% of
the U.S. population to over 30%. In the same time period, the percentage of poor individuals (under $15,000 a year in inflation-adjusted 1990 constant dollars) has risen
from 13.9% to 17%. Together, these groups represent a 14% decrease of the middle class
in its broadest definition. Miller speculates that there are three classes in the United
States, each comprising approximately one-third of the population: the struggling sector
(poverty and near it, including the working poor); the middle class; and the upscale
sector (both the affluent and those with appreciable amounts of discretionary income).

culture as is the middle class, but by earning enough to provide the basic comforts offered within a given society.

The lower-class role is determined in large part by birth, culture, and race. Some choose the role of poverty for specific moral and philosophical purposes; such as individuals are best exemplified by the spiritual leaders Jesus Christ, St. Francis of Assisi, Buddha, Mohammed, and (in modern times) Mohandas Gandhi. But most often poverty, as an accident of birth, functions as a means of repression and humiliation.

The Pariah

There may well be a fifth class, that of the pariah or outcast, who may belong to any economic class. Within a repressive society, the pariah may serve a political function, openly criticizing a government intent to silence any opposition. The intellectuals Andrei Sakharov and Alexander Solzhenitsyn are but two examples of pariah figures who served such a function in the former Soviet Union. Artists living within repressive countries have often taken on pariah roles and offered an oblique critique. Some pariahs, like Nelson Mandela, have lived to see a revolutionary political change that has led to their transformation from pariah to hero, or even, as in the case of the Czech playwright Vaclav Havel, from pariah to ruler.

There are many other types of pariahs with considerably diminished status. They include criminals, addicts, ethnic minorities, the mentally and terminally ill, elderly people, people with AIDS, homeless people, and deformed people, among others. These types of pariahs reveal the underside of a community. They serve as a reminder that on the other side of health, wealth, youth, security, and morality is a set of roles that not only exists within us all, but can surface without much warning. By casting them off and locking them away, we may believe that we are protecting ourselves from their immediate presence; however, we are not protected from their imagery, which we voraciously devour in the media and revisit in our nightmares.

Work Roles

In contrast to the pariah role are the work/occupational roles that for the most part serve to connect people to their communities. A given community will ascribe a status to each work role, which will vary according to time and place. An agrarian society will value its farmers; a technocracy will afford them scant attention. The kinds of work roles available vary considerably in the status, socioeconomic benefits, and degree of satisfaction they provide.

Individuals also vary in terms of their relationship to their work roles. For some, one occupational role is insufficient or limited in itself. William Carlos Williams, one of the great modern American poets, earned his living primarily as a doctor; one of his contemporaries, Wallace Stevens, was an insurance executive. Others change careers at midstream after experiencing a degree of burnout or boredom. Still others will continue to play out an unsatisfactory occupational role, justifying themselves with the argument of security while secretly dreaming, Walter Mitty-like, of assuming more exciting roles.

It could well be that our internalized cast of occupational roles affects not only our behavior, but also our ways of thinking about ourselves. For example, I see myself as technically incompetent and tend to freeze up when confronted with a stalled car or temperamental computer. It may be that I lack a certain mechanical aptitude, and because of that have avoided contact with mechanically oriented individuals as role models.

The full internal cast of occupational roles probably indicates the complexity and potential of human beings more clearly than the one or two work roles they play out in everyday life. To the extent that I can be more than a teacher, I will be able to live a full and rich work life, with minimal fear of burnout and workaholism. Work roles may appear to be primary, in the sense that traditional families of tailors, shoemakers, farmers, lawyers, and doctors, for example, tend to pass on their trades. Yet as one takes on further possibilities from the larger social/cultural world, more choices become available. And in playing out these possibilities vocationally and avocationally, individuals expand their sense of well-being. Even though I may never be able to fix my car, the possibility of mechanical success is very tantalizing. But before I get my hands to work, I need an image of myself as one who is able to work a machine. Without an appropriate role model, I give in to my somatic limitations and give over more power to machines then they deserve.

Authority and Power Roles

Finally, there is a class of social/cultural roles that in many ways applies to all of the others mentioned above. These roles concern authority and power. They may be viewed as existing along a continuum from passive to aggressive.

The passive one tends to retreat from social intercourse for many reasons, such as lack of interest, fear of engagement, maintenance of power, or control. The passive role can thus be weak or strong in quality. When weak, the passive one is unseen and perhaps neglected by others; furthermore, the weak passive one becomes easy prey to the aggressor and bully. When strong, one who practices passive resistance as a political act can greatly influence a society. Examples include Mohandas Gandhi and Martin Luther King, Jr., both of whom were instrumental in transforming their reigning political orders through nonviolent actions.

The aggressor as a role type can be seen in terms of opposing moral qualities. At its most negative, aggression is the use of force to assert one's power over those who do not willingly comply. Examples of negative aggressors include the tyrant and dictator, the bully, the sadist, the killer, and the abusive parent. Sometimes aggression is turned upon oneself, leading to the playing out of the masochist role or, in the extreme, that of the suicide.

Aggression also has a positive side, exemplified in the warrior role. Rather than usurping power or giving it up, warriors fight for a principle. The power of the warrior is as often intellectual and moral as physical. The battle to be won is generally internal, as warriors fight their own passive, conservative tendencies. Yet the warrior also competes with external enemies, negotiating with and confronting those authority figures who attempt to diminish their power. Children are warriors when they test out the power of their parents; parents are warriors when they set limits upon their children. Scholars are warriors when they dare to move beyond an accepted theory. Lawyers are warriors when they argue a case based upon principle. Addicts are warriors when they confront their disease and seek treatment. The warrior role can be the force that keeps those alive who feel most oppressed and hopeless.

It may be that we inherit a tendency to play out our authority roles in certain benevolent or malevolent ways. But even so, the role models we choose to follow, like the posters and photographs adolescents hang on their walls, will tell us at least as much about the ways we play out our authority on the streets where we walk and in the homes where we live.

SPIRITUAL ROLES

The conflict between the individual spiritual consciousness and the collective, often bureaucratic will of the church or other religious body has been a repeated theme in literature and history. The story of Joan of Arc has exemplified this theme since the Middle Ages. Saint Joan embodies a spiritual role—that of the visionary, a particular kind of believer. This role may be fully embraced or may become the source of internal conflict. What if Joan were uncertain that her visions were indeed holy ones? What if Christ doubted his divinity or chose to live a more conventional life—a situation envisioned in Nikos Kazantzakis's novel (1951/1961) and Martin Scorsese's film (1988), *The Last Temptation of Christ*? These kinds of questions are also germane to less saintly beings in everyday life wrestling with their own conflicts between faith and doubt.

From the point of view of society, the visionary is quite suspect. People who tend to have visions of God are generally thought to be delusional or mentally ill. A great cynicism in regard to the visionary role exists in most technologically advanced societies. In the United States, visionaries tend to achieve notoriety only when they commit a particular atrocity. Examples include the serial killer David Berkowitz, dubbed the Son of Sam, who claimed that his visions of destruction were dictated by a dog; and Charles Manson, the charismatic mass murderer who persuaded a group of stoned, lost disciples that his vision of Armageddon was near.

The role of visionary can, however, serve a significant function in our everyday lives. The visionary role may well be essential to the creative artist or scientist who is able to see through the veil of the everyday and expected, if only for a moment; with that insight, the visionary may develop a unique assessment or synthesis. But the visionary role is not the exclusive property of Copernicus and Newton, Shakespeare and Mozart, Einstein and Freud. It is part of us all when we are able to imagine a new order, a sense of how things might be. The role of visionary is not necessarily taken on to control external events, but to temper internal ones. That is, visionaries are in-sightful, turning their view inward in order to make sense of the empirical world. Many who take on the role of visionary may not actually choose to do so, but feel compelled to see in this way, as if called out by the role.

At some point in our lives, we may want more than vision; we may desire transcendence. Like Faust, we may be willing to pay a very high price indeed for transcendent knowledge or power. In doing so, we take on the powerful role of God in an attempt to control natural events ordinarily beyond our control. As such, we may indulge in the ecstasy of Dionysus, the prophecy of Apollo, the omnipotence and magnificent rage of Zeus, the wisdom of Athena, the beauty of Aphrodite, the forgiveness and love of Christ. Or we may shift into a more demonic role, playing Satan, Fury, or witch to express the fearful, dreadful impulses that often remain frozen for fear of being judged too harshly.

This urge for the transcendence of the gods and demons, or even the playfulness and delicacy of the sprites, can serve a very significant function in the earth-bound lives of most, especially those who have rejected a traditional view of religion. To play God may provide a needed expression of creativity and playfulness that affords a respite from the ordinariness of daily life. To play the being who is in control of that which is out of control temporarily relieves us of the need to control everything. It assures us that the intuitive, irrational, playful parts of ourselves are intact, even if for a moment, and that, as Hamlet says (Act I, scene v, 166–167),

> There are more things in heaven and earth, Horatio,
> Than are dreamt of in your philosophy.

Spiritual roles in relation to one's belief in religions or gods can be categorized as follows: orthodox believer, agnostic, atheist, and nihilist. Orthodox believers are committed fully to their faith. Agnostics are uncertain as to their belief in a given god. Atheists are certain that they do not believe in a religious deity, although they may choose a scientific, political, or aesthetic object of reverence. Nihilists deny the existence of all gods and all purpose in the universe. Belief systems develop much as moral roles do, through a combination of primary, secondary, and tertiary experiences in role.

There may be a generalized spiritual role that applies to believers, agnostics, and atheists alike, based on a search for meaning within existence. In mythology, anthropology, popular culture, and drama, this is the role of the hero. Heroes, also known as searchers, take a journey—whether a literal journeying forth into the world, or a voyage deep within the internalized role system in order to make sense of their existence. The heroic journey involves a confrontation with significant dangers and threats on both a psychological and a physical level. As such, the hero role is different from those roles associated with work, politics, morality, family, gender, and health; yet it is a part of all roles when one searches for the meaning within.

Heroic role models are needed in all cultures in order to provide individuals with a sense of perfectibility and possibility. The exploits of heroes are recapitulated in the play and fantasy of children and adolescents, as well as in the desires of adults for great wisdom and power.

Because we are living in an unheroic age, it may be argued, we look more to the antihero as a role model. The antihero is an ordinary person who struggles with ordinary problems, like Sam making out his will (see Chapter Two). Some turn radically to the negativity of the nihilist role, to remind themselves that the attempt to play the hero in the face of the meaninglessness of the journey is futile. Their evidence includes such cultural phenomena as the worldwide rise of the skinhead and neo-Fascist movements. The denial of meaning and purpose can serve a purposeful function for those who can channel their nihilism into appropriate postmodern art forms that demolish or deconstruct conventional notions of performance, text, movement, and music.

As one moves toward nonbeing and denies the searcher role, however, one gets closer to the realm of the zombie or suicide. Many suicides are dreamed about or planned; few are executed. To be or not to be—that is Hamlet's question. It is also ours when we have slipped into the roles of antihero and nihilist. To be or not to be what? Alive? Dead? One answer is heroic. The nonheroic life is a deadening one. To be heroic is to try to discover a way to make sense of our lives, whether we do it from the point of view of a god or a demon, of a superwoman or a low man, of an orthodox or a nihilist. As mentioned above, life in role is not an either–or proposition. It is a paradox, being and nonbeing existing side by side. When one takes on the role of hero—trying to discover, for example, how to assert authority in the face of an abusive, threatening power—there is always the possibility of being overcome not only by that power, but by one's own self-doubts as to one's right to fight. If one retreats because of such doubts, he has responded to Hamlet's question: Not to be, that is the answer. If one chooses to fight, he has transformed Hamlet's question into an answer, living not in the world of either–or, but of both–and. That is the domain of the hero.

AESTHETIC ROLES

Spiritual roles of the epic dimension often intersect with aesthetic roles, those pertaining to the creative process. The most significant aesthetic role, that of the artist, can also be seen as a hero and visionary role: The artist journeys into the world or the mind in order to discover some essential truths.

Visual, dance, and musical artists communicate their discoveries through images and shapes, movement and rhythm, sound and time—forms that communicate to an audience through the senses. These forms, while not the same as role, perhaps serve a similar purpose within the respective arts: to contain certain essential qualities unique to those arts. Dramatic and literary artists deal more directly with role through verbal language. Their creative process is one of a projection, imposing their visions and images upon fictional characters who are both similar to and different from the artists.

The role of the artist as creator is similar to that of God, the creator. Both bring forth life from nonlife, imagery from emptiness, order from chaos. Within many religious traditions, the artist metaphor is applied to God: God is poet, one who creates a language to name the things of creation; God is sculptor, molding human beings from clay; God is muse and impresario, inspiring creative activity; and God is dancer.

The role of creator demands attention to an unnameable, intuitive part of the personality. To create, one must be able to transcend the expected and the ordinary, or to enter the expected and ordinary as if seeing it for the first time. The creator role is thus full of possibility. It is a playful role, characterized by others as one of "flow" (see Csikszentmihalyi, 1990), "spontaneity" (see Moreno, 1946), "aesthetic distance" (see Scheff, 1979), "peak experience" (see Maslow, 1971), and "liminality" (see Turner, 1982).

The creative artist is one form of the creator role. All acts of everyday life can be performed creatively, just as all daily acts can be performed devoutly. When one takes on the creator role, one ceases to use expected language and gesture. One shifts into the space between the ordinary and the extraordinary. Within the creator role, one can discover meaning in the simplest act and, for a fraction of a second, feel fully alive.

Aesthetic roles, however, tend to be short-lived, operating according to Thomas Edison's antiromantic equation attributing 1% of creative genius to inspiration and 99% to perspiration. All working artists know the drudgery of the extended creative process. And the dreamer, another type that subsists within the aesthetic domain, knows too that he must soon abandon his romantic visions and return to the ground of the everyday. But without the creative moments life would be unbearable for many. One reason why human beings need gods in their lives as role models is to continue to be able to play out the role of God the creator. Many of the greatest artists of the 20th century have presented a godless universe ruled by the Beckett aphorism "Nothing to be done" (see *Waiting for Godot,* 1954). Yet people like Samuel Beckett and Ingmar Bergman have never ceased to embrace the role of the creator, perhaps the single most important part of their psyches.

It may well be that the great artists are born with their creative roles intact. But our role models need not be Michelangelo and Martha Graham. The creative role can be taken on from those who simply approach the tasks of everyday life with a degree of playfulness and spontaneity.

CHAPTER EIGHT

A Taxonomy of Roles:
Building a Theatrical
Archetype System

In building a theatrical archetype system, my aim is to establish connections among repeated role types and to uncover in theatrical form
a system of making sense of the complexities of existence as they are
revealed through character. This system draws upon many of the
categories and types delineated in the preceding chapter. My specific
concern is with identifying those role types that recur throughout
the history of Western theatre. To accommodate the complexity of
such broad role types as mother and wife, fool and hero, many types
are further subdivided.

A complete understanding of repeated role types entails a comprehensive review of theatre history. Others have successfully completed that task (see Brockett, 1990); their work might well serve as
a full reference. As context for particular role types, I offer examples
of characters from several different periods in theatre history (when
appropriate) to demonstrate the continuity of role types.

THE FORM OF THE TAXONOMY

The taxonomy that I present in the following four chapters offers a
reductionist approach to classifying the characters found within
Western dramatic literature. From this material I glean a series of role
types, which are prototypical forms implicit within the characters and
related to similar characters in dramatic literature. The taxonomy is
presented in eight parts:

1. Domains
2. Classifications within the domains
3. Role type
4. Subtype
5. Quality
6. Function
7. Style
8. Theatrical examples

Domains

Domains are the broadest categories of role, representing faculties of the human being. Consistent with the my discussion in Chapter Seven, I offer six domains:

1. Somatic—that which pertains to one's developmental, sexual, and physical aspects.
2. Cognitive—that which pertains to one's thinking style.
3. Affective—that which pertains to morality and feeling states.
4. Social—that which includes political and socioeconomic status, position within the family, and authority and power.
5. Spiritual—that which pertains to one's search for meaning and relationship with a transcendent being or transcendent part of oneself.
6. Aesthetic—that which pertains to the creative, artistic part of the human personality.

Classifications within the Domains

Classifications are subdivisions of domains that contain a related group of role types. The somatic domain, for example, is subdivided into the following classifications: age, sexual orientation, appearance, and health. Those classifications discussed in Chapter Seven that are too general in terms of theatrical role types (e.g., gender) are omitted from the taxonomy. Some domains are not subdivided into classifications because the specified role types are limited in quantity and clearly interrelated in substance. Within the cognitive domain, for example, I identify only five role types: the simpleton, the fool, the ambivalent one, the critic, and the wise one. Because all are interrelated, there is no need to subdivide this domain further.

The affective domain, on the other hand, contains two classifications. The first, concerning moral types, encompasses 15 specific roles—the greatest number given within any single classification of the taxonomy. It may well be that morality more than any other faculty drives theatrical characters. The second classification within the affective domain concerns feeling states, which correspond generally to a range of emotion from superrational, overdistanced, and dispassionate to irrational, underdistanced, and ecstatic.

The social domain encompasses the most role types of all, 33. These types are subdivided into five classifications: family, politics/government, legal, socioeconomic status, and authority and power. Work roles are omitted because they are too general.

The spiritual domain contains two classifications: natural beings and supernatural beings. Although this domain only encompasses 10 role types, it is significant in holding perhaps the most prominent dramatic and mythological role, the hero.

The final domain, that of the aesthetic, contains just two role types and is therefore devoid of classifications.

In chart form, the domains with their classifications appear as follows:

DOMAIN: SOMATIC

Classification: AGE
Classification: SEXUAL ORIENTATION
Classification: APPEARANCE
Classification: HEALTH

DOMAIN: COGNITIVE

DOMAIN: AFFECTIVE

Classification: MORAL
Classification: FEELING STATES

DOMAIN: SOCIAL

Classification: FAMILY
Classification: POLITICS/GOVERNMENT
Classification: LEGAL
Classification: SOCIOECONOMIC STATUS
Classification: AUTHORITY AND POWER

DOMAIN: SPIRITUAL

Classification: NATURAL BEINGS
Classification: SUPERNATURAL BEINGS

DOMAIN: AESTHETIC

Role Type

Each role type provides a meaningful constellation of related qualities. It presents archetypal rather than stereotypical qualities of a role. There have been a number of attempts to specify role types by psychologists and mythologists who, like Jung, focus upon archetypes derived from mythology. Pearson (1989), for example, specifies six role types: innocent, orphan, wanderer, warrior, martyr, and magician. Another attempt (Riso, 1987) is based in an ancient mystical diagram, the enneagram, and specifies nine role types: helper, status seeker, artist, thinker, loyalist, generalist, leader, peacemaker, and reformer.

Some involved in treating alcoholic families have conceived of role types representative of family dynamics, including the enabler, the hero, the scapegoat, the lost child, and the clown (see Kritsberg, 1988). Others working within the structural system of transactional analysis (see Berne, 1961), have identified three ego states equivalent to role types: Parent, Adult, and Child. Within the field of literary criticism, Propp (1968) has isolated types that appear in Russian folk tales, including hero, false hero, villain, dispatcher, helper, donor, princess, and father.

Focusing upon theatre, and tempering this focus with my study of repeated types in everyday life, I identify 84 role types, all organized within their domains and (when relevant) classifications. My study begins with the early Greek plays of Aeschylus and proceeds through contemporary Western forms of drama. This study is limited to a critical reading of approximately 600 plays—those that are frequently anthologized, summarized, and critiqued (see, e.g., Brockett, 1990; Gassner, 1954; Shipley, 1984; and Southern, 1961), and those that are regularly reviewed in such publications as *The Drama Review, Theatre Journal,* and *The New York Times.* In reviewing the many plays given in these and related sources, I have abstracted the role types that reappear throughout time and genre.

All characters in theatre are types to a certain extent. Some, like a moral virtue in a medieval morality play or a stock character in an Italian *commedia dell'arte,* are literal and simplistic, appearing to be fully equivalent to a role type. Examples include the cowardly soldier, the miserly father, the cuckolded husband, the wise servant, and the romantic lovers. Others, like Antigone, Hamlet, Blanche DuBois, and Willy Loman, are multidimensional, rich, and complex. It becomes clear that the character of Hamlet, for example, encompasses several role types: actor and scholar, lover and avenger, hero and fool. Yet even Hamlet and related complex characters are abstractions of the human spirit—less stereotypical than characters in a morality play, but types nonetheless, whether prototypical tragic heroes or modern realistic antiheroes.

A role type, then, can be one part of a dramatic character who also embodies other role types, or a whole character who is drawn broadly and simply. To the extent that theatrical role type and character are one, the dramatic function will remain rather simple, and the style of enactment will tend to be broad and larger than life. To the extent that the character embodies many role types, as Hamlet and Antigone do, the functions will need to be specified for each, and the style will tend more toward the representational. As characters become more complex, then, they approach the actual status of human beings.

On the other hand, it may also be true that the more a playwright is able to chip a character down to certain essential and simple qualities, such as the naiveté and absurdity of Bottom in Shakespeare's *A Midsummer Night's Dream,* the more he creates a clearly discerned form that may well recapitulate the experience of many viewers. Perhaps this is a major function of role in theatre—to endow a character with such particular nuance; to discover small, personal, human ways to fill large, abstract, conceptual masks so that an audience can respond by saying: "Yes, we too see some truth about our own experience in that role!"

The relationship between role type and complex character is a paradoxical one. On the one hand, as noted above, complexity leads to a representational style approaching the real life of a human being. On the other, simplicity, the small, well-observed movements of a stock character type, leads to a complex understanding of human behavior—a thought expressed by the poet William Blake as envisioning the world in a grain of sand (see *Auguries of Innocence,* 1790/1964). Blake's vision might well have been shared by the great playwrights, like Shakespeare and Molière, whose simple role types moved toward complexity and whose complex characters, in the elegant unfolding of their parts, offered both a human and a cosmic simplicity.

Subtype

Subtype is a further division of role type, useful in classifying variations on a similar theme or alternative qualities of the same type. For example, the fool type can generate such subtypes as the trickster and the existential clown. Although these are variations on the fool type, each one implies a somewhat unique quality, function, and/or style, given the fact that it exists within its own particular genre and historical moment.

As another example, several alternative qualities of the mother as primary role type are found in dramatic literature. When there is a powerful contrast to the nurturing mother, such as the murderous mother, a subtype is be specified.

Quality

Quality is a description of the role type or subtype, including physical, cognitive, moral, emotional, social, and spiritual aspects of the role. Characters of similar type (or subtype) have similar qualities that are derived from an analysis of their behavior and motivations within dramatic literature. Typical villains—Creon and Iago, for example—all tend to exemplify the same need for power and control. Complex role types present diverse and often contradictory qualities. Iago, as classical villain, is both invulnerable and vulnerable, both trusted and reviled, of high intelligence yet low motives; in many ways he is like Milton's Satan in *Paradise Lost* (1667/1957), one who aspires to playing God. Yet even so, the links among those of a similar type are established by a common set of descriptors as well as a shared dramatic function. When contrasting qualities are highly contradictory, a subtype is established.

Function

Function addresses the purpose of a particular role within the context of the play as well as the relationship between a role type and an audience. Propp (1968), who (as noted above) taxonomized qualities of plot and character in more than 100 Russian folk tales, defined character function as "an act of character defined from the point of view of its significance for the course of the action" (p. 21). This is similar to my conception of role function, but I also assume a theatrical sense of function. Thus, each role serves a particular function within the mind of a character and text of a play, and it is the actor's job to discover that function and communicate it to an audience. Although a role may serve some contradictory functions within a drama, there still remains a primary motivation or spine that provides each role type with a sense of purpose. All fools, for example, may not express their wit and wisdom in a similar fashion. Yet they all function generally to offer their foolish wisdom to those willing to listen or foolish enough to turn a deaf ear. In relation to an audience, the fool may serve various functions, according to individuals' needs. However, most audience members will be able to view their own real-life foolishness from a distance in identifying with the role type on stage.

Style

The degree of identification between role type and audience will be determined to a great extent by the style of production. Style is the behavioral form in which the role is enacted, whether reality-based and representational, abstract and presentational, or somewhere in between. Each style implies a specified degree of affect and cognition. The representational style implies a greater degree of emotion; the presentational a greater degree of cognition. As such, style in theatre operates in ways that are similar to the distancing model mentioned above. The overdistanced position, characterized by an abundance of cognition and a modicum of affect, is operative within more presentational styles of performance. The underdistanced position, with its excess of affect and dearth of cognition, reflects more representational styles.

Style, in many ways, determines behavior and level of emotional expression. Yet, although certain genres of theatre point to certain given styles, the actor and director may choose to work against that style to some degree in order to depict a complex character who is both abstract and real, universal condition and specific case.

I generally allot a specific style to a role type when that role seems historically and aesthetically married to that style; for example, the existential clown of Beckett's plays is unmistakably presentational. In many other cases, when I assume that the role type can easily be enacted in both styles, I omit a specific notation of style.

Theatrical Examples

Examples are provided from at least three different periods/genres in theatre history when relevant (e.g., classical Greek and Roman, Renaissance, and modern). This point substantiates, in part, the universal nature of the role types. Some role types tend to be specific to a certain historical period, such as the modern and postmodern antihero. In such cases, I provide examples from diverse plays written within that period. However, most of the 84 role types delineated are seen as recurring throughout time, place, and genre.

THE TAXONOMY OF ROLES

The full taxonomy is presented below and continues through Chapter Eleven.

DOMAIN: SOMATIC

Classification: AGE

I. Role Type: Child

   Quality: The child is playful, fun-loving, egocentric, and guileless. This role type most often is that of a preadolescent who behaves in a manner consistent with these qualities. In some cases, older characters present themselves in a childlike manner and thus embody aspects of this role type.
   Function: The function of the child is to assert the playful spirit, innocence, and wonder of childhood.
   Style: In many ways, this is a romanticized notion of childhood, which implies a presentational form of performance. The vast majority of child characters remain consistent to this view and thus appear on the stage as less than realistic. Yet many of the child characters who appear in plays call for a mixture of styles, as is the case in high-quality children's theatre scripts that address contemporary social or psychological issues (see, e.g., S. Zeder's *Step on a Crack* and W. Kesselman's *Maggie, Magalita*).
   Examples: The role type of the child has appeared at least since the early Greek tragedies and comedies in a simplified form. From the Renaissance to the present, the child role type expanded in complexity and began to appear with some frequency. The prototypical child role, Peter Pan, is most characteristic of this type, and has been the source of endless theatrical productions and social and psychological speculations.
   The following examples begin in the late 16th century, spanning a number of centuries and genres: Edward III (*Edward II* by C. Marlowe), The Child (*Woyzeck* by G. Büchner), Little Eva (*Uncle Tom's Cabin*, adaptation of H. B. Stowe novel by G. Aiken), Hedwig (*The Wild Duck* by H. Ibsen), Tyltyl and Mytil (*The Blue Bird* by M. Maeterlinck), Hannele (*Hannele* by G. Hauptmann), Trouble (*Madame Butterfly* by D. Belasco), Peter Pan (*Peter Pan* by J. M. Barrie), and Annie (*Annie* by T. Mahan, C. Strouse, and M. Charnin).

2. Role Type: Adolescent

Quality: The adolescent is self-conscious, moral and righteous, searching, sentimental and romantic, and naive and awkward. Although the age ranges within the teen years, adolescent qualities also apply to adult characters.

Function: Adolescence is a transitional period between childhood and adulthood. As a role type, the adolescent functions to demonstrate the comic and tragic consequences of living in a psychological stage of being that is neither innocent nor experienced.

Style: This role type, though easily satirized and given to stylized forms of performance, has become more representational in the work of modern playwrights such as Tennessee Williams and Peter Shaffer.

Examples: Shakespeare presents a rich array of adolescent characters, most notably Romeo and Juliet. Strong examples from the 19th and 20th centuries include Melchior and Wendla (*Spring's Awakening* by F. Wedekind), Nina (*The Sea Gull* by A. Chekhov), Wendy (*Peter Pan* by J. M. Barrie), Richard Miller *Ah, Wilderness!* by E. O'Neill), Dorothy (*The Wizard of Oz* by L. F. Baum), Laura (*The Glass Menagerie* by T. Williams), Alan Strang (*Equus* by P. Shaffer), and Mozart (*Amadeus* by P. Shaffer)

3. Role Type: Adult

Quality: As a role type, the adult is responsible, committed, rational, dependable, and strong, yet vulnerable. The adult figure is not tied to any set age or gender, but is one who inspires trust.

Function: The adult functions as a balancer, an often moral figure offering stability and reason to those less stable and less reasonable.

Style: Many adult figures, especially from the 20th century, are drawn in a realistic way, although certain classical examples, given the nature of the genres in which they appear, are intended to be played more presentationally.

Examples: Exemplary adult figures include the following: Theseus (*Oedipus at Colonus* by Sophocles), The Nurse (*Romeo and Juliet* by Shakespeare), Mr. and Mrs. Darling (*Peter Pan* by J. Barrie), Atticus Finch (*To Kill a Mockingbird,* adaptation of H. Lee novel by H. Foote), Big Daddy (*Cat on a Hot Tin Roof* by T. Williams), and Lieutenant Ralph Clark (*Our Country's Good* by T. Wertenbaker).

4. Role Type: Elder (see also Grandparent)

Quality: The elder is wise, philosophical, prophetic, and sympathetic. Although young characters sometimes possess these qualities, the role type is generally reserved for one of senior citizen status. The elder is sometimes eccentric, like Grandpa Vanderhof (*You Can't Take It with You* by G. Kaufman and M. Hart).

Function: The elder functions to pass on to the younger generation the wisdom acquired through age and experience. Elders also exhibit the charming eccentricities often associated with age.

Style: The wise, philosophical elder tends to be enacted in a realistic style.

Examples: Gonzalo (*The Tempest* by Shakespeare), Countess of Rossillion (*All's Well That Ends Well* by Shakespeare), Captain Shotover (*Heartbreak House* by G. B. Shaw), Jacob (*Awake and Sing* by C. Odets), Abby and Martha Brewster (*Arsenic and Old Lace* by J. Kesselring), Hugh (*Translations* by B. Friel), and Emil and George (*Duck Variations* by D. Mamet).

4.1. Subtype: Lecher

Quality: Elders may also appear irascible, lecherous, controlling, egocentric, and foolish.

Function: These elders covet and/or attempt to control the young, often making fools of themselves in the process.

Style: The lecherous variety of elder is generally enacted in a presentational style.

Examples: The alternative form of the elder was prevalent in classical drama, especially in the Roman comedies. This elder also became popular with the character of Pantalone in the Renaissance *commedia dell'arte*. Specific examples include Old Lysidamus (*Casina* by Plautus), Sir Toby Belch (*Twelfth Night* by Shakespeare), Husband/Boss (*Machinal* by S. Treadwell), and Max (*The Homecoming* by H. Pinter).

Classification: SEXUAL ORIENTATION

5. Role Type: Eunuch

Quality: The eunuch is one who is asexual—castrated and impotent. Eunuchs are generally sexually ambiguous and appear paradoxical in being both threatening to and trusted by those who are sexually insecure. Furthermore, they are often verbal and witty, sometimes light and comic, other times pathetic.

Function: The eunuch provides audiences members a chance to release castration anxieties through laughter. The role type performs the paradoxical function of threatening and mollifying the threats to sexually insecure individuals.

Style: This character, appearing most frequently in classical Roman drama and Renaissance drama, was generally drawn in broad strokes and highly stylized. In its modern incarnations, it tends to be more humanly drawn and thus enacted with greater emotional investment, as exemplified by the character Brick (*Cat on a Hot Tin Roof* by T. Williams). Some audience members may harbor dimly realized fears of sexual inadequacy. Through the often stylized, sexually charged issues raised by the presence of the eunuch, they are in essence given permission to laugh at their own sexual fears in a safe way.

Examples: Examples from classical, modern, and contemporary drama include The Eunuch (*The Eunuch* by Terence), Lucrezia (*Mandragola* by N. Machiavelli), Castrone (*Volpone* by B. Jonson), Alexas (*All for Love* by J. Dryden), Acmat (*The Royal Mischief* by M. D. Manley), Two Eunuchs (*The Visit* by F. Dürrenmatt), Pothinus (*Caesar and Cleopatra* by G. B. Shaw), Hinkemann (*Hinkemann* by E. Toller), and La Zambinella (*Sarrasine* by N. Bartlett).

6. Role Type: Homosexual

Quality: One version of this role type offers the qualities of sensitivity and wit, vulnerability, and the expression of passionate feelings. The homosexual tends to be an outsider, yet in many ways fights for acceptance—if not in the mainstream, at least within a community of peers. The gay character is also dramatized as insecure, angry and hostile, bitchy and decadent.

Function: The gay role type challenges conventional sexual morality, sometimes raging against the homophobia of the straight world. This role type also offers an alternative lifestyle.

Style: In *Edward II* by C. Marlowe, Edward's love for the opportunist, Gaveston, is portrayed in a harsh political light because it motivates the nobles of the court to revolt against their king, leading to the brutal execution of Edward. This relationship is a far cry from the idyllic romps between older men and young boys occasionally alluded to in the comedies of Aristophanes.

The role type of homosexual has evolved considerably in recent times. The mid-20th-century theatre presented a more personal view of a vulnerable pariah, alternatively angry, bitchy, and gentle. In the age of AIDS, the role type has again shifted from the personal to the political realm in plays where the victimized pariah must express his anger and his revolutionary spirit in order to influence the conventional order. As with other sexual role types, the homosexual is often portrayed as larger than life and thus presentational. However, in that most of the examples are recent, the trend has been toward more realistic depictions of character.

Examples: Although portrayed throughout theatre history, the homosexual character has achieved its fullest status as a major role type in modern and contemporary theatre. The first developed gay character, Gaveston in *Edward II* (see above), appeared in the Renaissance. More modern examples include: Countess Geschwitz (*Pandora's Box* by F. Wedekind), Inez (*No Exit* by J.-P. Sartre), Christopher (*I Am A Camera* by J. Van Druten), Martha Dobie (*The Children's Hour* by L. Hellman), Alfred Redl (*A Patriot for Me* by J. Osborne), Geoffrey (*A Taste of Honey* by S. Delaney), June (*The Killing of Sister George* by F. Marcus), Lin (*Cloud Nine* by C. Churchill), Max (*Bent* by M. Sherman), Kenny (*The Fifth of July* by L. Wilson), Rich and Saul (*As If* by W. Hoffman), and Ed (*Torch Song Trilogy* by H. Fierstein).

7. Role Type: Transvestite

Quality: The transvestite is a cross-dresser, often campy, amoral, outrageous, and unconventional. This character type is often highly verbal, witty, and creative.

Function: The transvestite functions to poke fun at conventional sexual morality and to celebrate the free expression of ambivalent sexuality.

Style: Although the transvestite is generally enacted in a presentational style, a less farcical view is presented in two contemporary plays by H. Fierstein, *La Cage aux Folles* and *Torch Song Trilogy*, where the protagonists as cross-dressers are depicted in a realistic fashion and thus establish a direct empathetic connection with the audience. In these examples, the transvestite role, although still that of a pariah, aspires to bourgeois status. This is very different from the more presentationally drawn, iconoclastic characters of C. Ludlam, who see themselves as functioning normally within a ridiculous universe. H. Fierstein's protagonist, Arnold, functions within a straight world; although he desires to remain gay, he aspires to social respectability.

Examples: Ben Jonson, a contemporary of Shakespeare, was a master of generating character types. An original Jonson creation in terms of role type is that of Epicene in the play of the same name, an androgynous character whose ambivalent sexuality serves to ridicule the pretensions of Old Morose, a hypochondriac and misogynist who will marry anybody as long as she is mute. The wife turns out to be a boy in drag, part of a scam arranged by Morose's nephew.

Epicene paves the way for more modern forms of sexual farce with characters in drag, such as the transvestite protagonist in C. Ludlam's *Camille,* who serves to poke fun at conventional sexual morality. A harsher version of sexual farce is found in the plays of J. Orton, whose *What the Butler Saw* presents an array of cross-dressing and cross-purposes. Further examples of the transvestite include: Rio Rita (*The Hostage* by B. Behan), Leslie Bright (*The Madness of Lady Bright* by L. Wilson), and Song Lilong (*M. Butterfly* by D. H. Hwang).

8. Role Type: Bisexual

Quality: The bisexual is one who is sexually attracted to members of both sexes. There is often an amoral quality within this role type.

Function: The bisexual functions, like the homosexual, to challenge conventional morality. This role further functions as a means of veiling the clear lines of sexual attraction between either opposite genders or similar genders. As such, the bisexual is a confusing role that may invoke a viewer's sexual ambivalence. On the other hand, the bisexual role may point to a healthy psychological androgyny, as suggested in the Jungian concepts of anima and animus.

Style: As in other cases of sexual roles, the bisexual often lends itself to presentational styles of enactment. However, within the more modern traditions, this role, like other sexual role types humanly drawn, can well be played realistically.

Examples: Realistic examples of bisexual characters have appeared in recent years in mainstream plays such as *Torch Song Trilogy* by H. Fierstein and *Falsettos* by W. Finn. In grappling with sexuality, playwrights have used this role as a means of exploring a primal conflict inherent within all human beings. The first example, notably, is of the god in whose name Greek drama was conceived—Dionysus, who has appeared in numerous classical and modern plays (e.g., *The Bacchae* by Euripides and *Dionysus in 69* by The Performance Group).

Other examples of the bisexual role type include Edward II (*Edward II* by C. Marlowe), Achilles (*Troilus and Cressida* by Shakespeare), Androgyno (*Volpone* by B. Jonson), Thérèse (*The Breasts of Tiresias* by G. Apollonaire), Nicholas Beckett (*What the Butler Saw* by J. Orton), and Victoria (*Cloud Nine* by C. Churchill).

Classification: APPEARANCE

9. Role Type: Beauty (see also Innocent and Immoralist)

Quality: This is the type of outstanding physical beauty in face and body, sometimes extending to a moral and spiritual quality. Beauty is an innocent in the fairy-tale sense.

Function: Beauty functions to dazzle and enchant. This type serves as an object of purity and/or love.

Style: In style, the beauty remains mostly presentational, as an ideal.

Examples: Examples include Iole (*The Women of Trachis* by Sophocles), Miranda (*The Tempest* by Shakespeare), Helen of Troy (*Doctor Faustus* by C. Marlowe), Mélisande (*Pélléas and Mélisande* by M. Maeterlinck), Deirdre (*Deirdre of the Sorrows* by J. M. Synge), and Maggie (*After the Fall* A. Miller).

9.1. Subtype: Seductress/Seducer

Quality: Beauty as seductress/seducer is experienced and calculating, using beauty as a means to satisfy her/his material and/or psychological needs.

Function: The calculating beauty seduces for her/his own selfish ends.

Style: Although this subtype can be performed in high style, it is often enacted representationally in modern drama.

Examples: Perhaps the most famous beauty in all mythology and drama is Helen of Troy, whose face launched a thousand ships. The innocent Helen is well represented by Marlowe's Renaissance version, referred to above. The calculating Helen is represented by Euripides's version in the play *Helen*. Other examples include Cleopatra (*Antony and Cleopatra* by Shakespeare), Carmen (*Carmen* by H. Meilhac and L. Halevy), and Lula (*The Dutchman* by A. Baraka).

10. Role Type: Beast (see also Physically Disabled and Demon)

Quality: The beast is the role of the ugly one, characterized by extremely unattractive looks in face and body, sometimes extending to a moral and/or spiritual quality.

Function: The function of the beast is to frighten and terrorize. On a more psychological level, the beast reveals the shadowy, dark side of human nature.

Style: The beast is generally portrayed in a stylized, dramatically compelling fashion.

Examples: The earliest beasts appeared in Greek drama as satyrs, comic contrivances that formed the basis of the satyr plays. These half-men, half-goats were generally bawdy and satirical, yet the one remaining satyr play, Euripides's *The Cyclops*, presents a more serious beast. Taken from Homer's *Odyssey*, The cyclops is an excellent example of the beast—a brutal giant with one eye who is capable of ripping trees out of the ground and eating men whole. Further examples include Caliban (*The Tempest* by Shakespeare), De Flores (*The Changeling* by T. Middleton and W. Rowley), Mr. Hyde (*Dr. Jekyll and Mr. Hyde*, adaptation of R. L. Stevenson novel by D. Edgar), and Leila (*The Screens* by J. Genet).

10.1. Subtype: Innocent Beast

Quality: Although physically ugly and/or frightening, this subtype of the beast possesses a spiritual innocence, often arousing sympathy and empathy.

Function: The innocent beast functions to exemplify the paradoxical relationship of body and spirit.

Examples: Lord Ravensbane (*The Scarecrow* by P. MacKaye), Frankenstein's monster (*Frankenstein*, adaption of M. Shelley novel by P. Webling), The Golem (*The Golem* by H. Leivik), Ivona (*Ivona, Princess of Burgundia* by W. Gombrowicz), Lenny (*Of Mice and Men* by J. Steinbeck), John Merrick (*The Elephant Man* by B. Pomerance), and Phantom (*The Phantom of the Opera* by R. Stilgoe and A. Lloyd Webber).

11. Role Type: Average One (see also Middle Class, Lost One, Everyman, and Antihero)

Quality: The average one is plain and nondescript, of ordinary appearance and stature, a nonentity, often alienated. Although ordinary, the average one occasionally becomes entangled within extraordinary circumstances.

Function: This role type functions to blend in, to look and behave like everyone else. The average one caught up in extraordinary circumstances expresses the malleability of human beings.

Style: The average one is, generally speaking, a modern character often played out in a minimal, absurdist style. Many modern exemplars have lost their names or taken on symbolic ones, such as Mr. Zero in E. Rice's *The Adding Machine*. Yet this type also appears more full-blown in realistic plays as an antihero, like Willy Loman in A. Miller's *Death of a Salesman* (see Chapter Eleven), who moves within a very limited psychological landscape.

Examples: Josef K. (*The Trial,* adaptation of F. Kafka novel by J. L. Barrault), Berenger (*The Killer* by E. Ionesco), Mommy and Daddy (*The American Dream* by E. Albee), Angel (*When You Coming Home, Red Ryder* by M. Medoff), and Garbagemen (*The Domestic Resurrection Circus* by P. Schumann). Examples of the average one caught up in extraordinary circumstances include: Galy Gay (*A Man's a Man* by B. Brecht), Johnny Johnson (*Johnny Johnson* by P. Green), Pantagleize (*Pantagleize* by M. de Ghelderode), and Anton Ignatyevich Kerzhentsev (*Poor Murderer* by P. Kohut).

Classification: HEALTH

12. Role Type: Mentally Ill/Mad Person

Quality: The mad person is unpredictable and irrational, manic and/or depressive, threatening to self or others.

Function: The mad person reveals the dark, shadowy sides of human nature and challenges the conventional notion of sanity. In part because of the audiences' needs to escape from the everyday and visit the dark recesses of madness vicariously, and in part because of their desire for a good scare, this stylized type has remained eminently popular throughout the centuries.

Style: In the Greek drama, we find a number of characters (e.g., Pentheus and the Furies) committing acts of madness under the Dionysian influence. As such, they are portrayed in a highly presentational manner. In Shakespeare's plays, the acts of madness are more clearly motivated by psychological factors. King Lear rages on the heath because he has allowed all his power to slip away and feels depleted of all sense of purpose. Lady Macbeth compulsively washes her hands because of the unbearable guilt she carries for her murderous act. For those driven mad by psychological factors, the enactment tends to become more representational.

Examples: As popular entertainment during the 18th century, some in the privileged classes would visit the madhouses for entertainment, a reality well depicted in the 20th-century play *Marat/Sade* by P. Weiss. And since the 1950s, a whole subgenre of horror films has developed concerning acts of violence committed by mad people. Other examples of this role type from classical and modern plays include: Ajax (*Ajax* by Sophocles), Henry IV (*Henry IV* by L. Pirandello), Mary Tyrone (*Long Day's Journey into Night* by E. O'Neill), Blanche DuBois (*A Streetcar Named Desire* by T. Williams), Captain Queeg (*The Caine Mutiny Court Martial* by H. Wouk), and Jack (*The Ruling Class* by P. Barnes).

13. Role Type: Physically Disabled or Deformed (see also Beast)

Quality: In quality, this type is frightening, unpredictable, and tempermental, either passive or aggressive. It is in many ways related to the beast type, described above. It is different in that it tends to be more often the misshapen human being and less often the science fiction monster.

Function: The functions of this type are to frighten; to play with the boundaries between the beautiful, the acceptable, and the ugly; and/or to act in such a way that the character's dark motivations reflect the misshapen appearance.

Style: The physically disabled is generally enacted within a presentational style.

Examples: Four character types appearing after 100 B.C. in Rome were credited to an ancient, nonscripted form of comedy, the Atellan farce, whose origins are unknown. The types include Bucco, a braggart warrior, Pappus, a comic old man; Maccus, a greedy fool; and Dossenus, a frightening-looking hunchback (see Brockett, 1990). The hunchback character, a precursor of Shakespeare's Richard III, is an early example of the physically disabled role type. More modern examples include Blind Man (*A Dream Play* by A. Strindberg), Bradley (*Buried Child* by S. Shepard), and Julia (*Fefu and Her Friends* by M. I. Fornes).

13.1. Subtype: Deformed as Transcendent

Quality: An alternative type of physical disability is that of the character who is moral, full of feeling, evocative of pathos, soulful, and powerful of stature.

Function: This type plays with the mythic and romantic notion that beauty of the spirit lives within a deformed appearance. The tragically heroic Oedipus is physically disabled, born with a clubfoot that provided his name. This quality of Oedipus points to a further dramatic function of the physically disabled—to suffer the rejection of others for an imperfection given at birth or acquired some time after. In coping with that rejection, one may choose (or be chosen) to follow the heroic path of Oedipus or the villainous one of Richard III.

Style: This alternative type tends more toward the representational, as it requires a more affective and affecting performance from an actor.

Examples: Gloucester (*King Lear* by Shakespeare), Porgy (*Porgy* by D. Heyward), Helen Keller (*The Miracle Worker* by W. Gibson), Sarah Norman (*Children of a Lesser God* by M. Medoff), and Ken Harrison (*Whose Life Is It Anyway?* by B. Clark).

14. Role Type: Hypochondriac

Quality: This type—obsessive, self-indulgent, foolish, insecure, and gullible—worries constantly about being sick.

Function: The hypochondriac strives to remain safe, protected from the imagined fears of illness and the world outside. If he is affluent, he may open himself up to quack doctors, suitors, and parasites waiting in the wings to serve him for their own personal gain. This role type often provides comic relief.

Style: The hypochondriac is generally a comic and foolish character, portrayed in a broad, presentational fashion.

Examples: In *The Imaginary Invalid,* Molière has created the classical hypochondriac, Argan, who exemplifies all of the above-described qualities. In modern drama, Chekhov has created an amusing representative, Lomov in *The Marriage Proposal.* There have been several musicals based upon Molière's *The Imaginary Invalid* including *Toinette* by J. Rodale and D. Meyer, and *Show Me Where the Good Times Are* by L. Thuna, K. Jacobson, and R. Roberts. In the latter, Argan becomes Aaron, a wealthy Lower East Side Jewish merchant; as in the Molière material, this character is used for farcical purposes. Other examples include Zeena (*Ethan Frome,* adaptation of E. Wharton novel by O. and D. Davis) and Felix (*The Odd Couple* by N. Simon).

15. Role Type: Doctor

Quality: The doctor is a healer of the body and soul. In its positive incarnation, this type is moral, dedicated, and competent.

Function: The function of the doctor is to help people by curing their ills, both physical and mental.

Examples: Doctors have appeared throughout the history of drama, although most of those who appeared in classical plays had minor roles. Examples include the doctors in *Everyman* by Anonymous and *King Lear* by Shakespeare. In modern and contemporary drama, the doctor role has become more prominent as healers themselves have assumed the status of tragic and comic protagonists. Examples include Dr. Astroff (*Uncle Vanya* by A. Chekhov), Colenso Ridgeon (*The Doctor's Dilemma* by G. B. Shaw), Dr. Hochberg (*Men in White* by S. Kingsley), Walter Reed (*Yellow Jack* by S. Howard), Dr. Dysart (*Equus* by P. Shaffer), and Hornby (*A Kind of Alaska* by H. Pinter).

15.1. Subtype: Quack Doctor

Quality: An ancient Roman comedy, *The Menaechmi* by Plautus, offers an early example of this figure who would become a stock character in later comedies. In quality, the quack doctor is arrogant, greedy, exploitative, pedantic, and silly.

Function: This type functions to use the powerful position of healer to exploit hypochondriacal or sick people in need of cures.

Style: Although a highly stylized character, the quack doctor is also found in more representational dramas, such as F. Dürrenmatt's *The Visit*.

Examples: Other examples of the quack doctor from various periods include Sgaranelle (*The Doctor in Spite of Himself* by Molière), Dr. Knock (*Doctor Knock* by J. Romains), and Dr. Prentice (*What the Butler Saw* by J. Orton). Broad portraits of the quack doctor were found in American burlesque and English music hall performances throughout the first half of the 20th century.

CHAPTER NINE

The Taxonomy:
Cognitive and
Affective Domains

DOMAIN: COGNITIVE

16. Role Type: Simpleton

Quality: The role type of the fool is often confused with that of the simpleton. The differences between the two are significant in that the fool is generally clever and witty, whereas the simpleton is naive and guileless, an easy target for ridicule. He is often ignorant and unaware of his ignorance; he is thus foolish without possessing the privileges and intelligence of the fool.

Function: The simpleton offers himself up for ridicule. He remains unaware and simple, no matter what the consequences.

Style: The simpleton is generally presented in a broad, presentational way.

Examples: Renaissance drama presents a wide array of simpletons, well exemplified by Bottom, the crass mechanical from Shakespeare's *A Midsummer Night's Dream,* who both literally and figuratively wears the head of an ass. The Italian *commedia dell'arte* often presented the simpleton as a servant, in contrast to such clever servants as Arlecchino.

Other examples throughout several periods in theatre history include Strepsiades (*The Clouds* by Aristophanes), Bartholomew Cokes (*Bartholomew Fair* by B. Jonson), King Peter of Popo (*Leonce and Lena* by G. Büchner), Judke (*The Treasure* by D. Pinski), Bob (*American Buffalo* by D. Mamet), and Lonnie Roy McNeill (*The Last Meeting of the Knights of the White Magnolia* by P. Jones).

16.1. Subtype: Cuckold

Quality: The cuckold is generally seen as naive and sexually incompetent. The cuckold exists as an object of humiliation, one who is made the fool by virtue of ignorance of his spouse's sexual escapades.

Function: The cuckold offers comic relief as he is humiliated upon discovering what others apparently know—that his spouse has been sexually unfaithful.

Style: The cuckold is generally presented in a broad style, with the exception of more contemporary plays (e.g., H. Pinter's *Betrayal*), where the cuckolded characters are realistically portrayed.

Examples: Amphitryon (*Amphitryon* by Plautus), The Husband (*Johan, Johan* by J. Heywood), Master Ford (*The Merry Wives of Windsor* by Shakespeare), Pinchwife (*The Country Wife* by W. Wycherley), Boubouroche (*Boubouroche* by G. Courteline), Bruno (*The Magnificent Cuckold* by F. Crommelynck), Casanova (*Camino Real* by T. Williams), and Max (*The Real Thing* by T. Stoppard).

17. Role Type: Fool

Quality: The role type of the fool extends from an early form of witty servant, first seen in the Greek comedies and highly visible in the Roman comedies. In quality, the witty servant and the later, more generic fool type both exist as foils to their unliberated, servile masters. The fool is subservient to the master, yet superior in wit and practical knowledge. This tends to be an ironic character who withholds knowledge from other characters, while sharing it with the audience. The fool's appeal is in superior awareness and ability to manipulate those of inferior intelligence. There is also a pathetic quality to the fool, since despite his wit he will remain lowly, perhaps unlovable, and socially unacceptable to his superiors.

Function: The function of the fool is to charm the master (and the audience) on the one hand, while offering up a critique of his foibles on the other. This lively character provides an alternative to the dullness of the master. The fool's low social status masks his high intelligence. There is a certain safety in his barbs and insights, in that he never has to be taken seriously because of his lowly social status. He establishes an empathetic bond with members of the audience, who, sharing in his privileged knowledge, desire to remain like him—superior in their own wisdom, though often at the expense of another.

Style: The fool is generally a highly stylized character, requiring a high degree of verbal dexterity and sleight of hand on the part of the actor.

Examples: The fool can be found prominently in early Roman comedy such as *Pseudolus* (represented by such characters as Plautus's Pseudolus); in Renaissance *commedia dell'arte,* and in many derivative productions, such as the musical comedy *A Funny Thing Happened on the Way to the Forum* by B. Shevelove, L. Gilbert, and S. Sondheim (where a similarly named Pseudolus holds forth). The prototype of the classical fool, derived in large part from the earlier witty servant, is embodied in the Italian Arlecchino, the comic trickster who is witty, wise, and mischievous. Arlecchino is often accompanied by the character Brighella, a cynical libertine with a decidedly cruel streak, more the rogue than the fool.

In later developments of the Arlecchino character, we find the fool, Pulcinella, an early version of the English puppet character Punch. This fool becomes a paradoxical character, embodying qualities of tenderness and deception, wisdom and ignorance, innocence and cunning. In Pulcinella, we begin to see the ambivalences of role quality that drive many of the most fully developed dramatic characters.

Shakespeare's Fool in *King Lear* is a sophisticated and complex version of these character types; although witty and ironic, he also takes on a certain human tragic dimension as he unwittingly gets caught up in the political events and is murdered. Shakespeare's fools come in many shapes and sizes, the roundest of which are the fully drawn Falstaff and Sir Toby Belch. Such fools have given birth to endless progeny, who include Truffaldino, the *commedia dell'arte*-like prankster in *The Servant of Two Masters* by C. Goldini; He, the pathetic clown in the abstract *He Who Gets Slapped* by L. Andreyev; the silly and sleepy Rip Van Winkle in the play of the same name (adaptation of W. Irving story by D. Boucicault); the ironic Herald in *Marat/Sade* by P. Weiss; and the androgynous and frightening Master of Ceremonies in *Cabaret* by J. Mastroff, J. Kander, and F. Ebb, among many others.

17.1. Subtype: Trickster (see also Fairy)

Quality: Originally a mythological character, the trickster is mischievous, amoral, and playful. Often androgynous and Dionysian in spirit, the trickster wreaks havoc with the lives of those who demand orderliness and efficiency.

Function: The trickster exists to transform the familiar into the strange and to shake up the expected, conventional order of things, causing discord and chaos (at least temporarily). This early version of the fool is devoted to mischief and anarchy.

Style: The trickster is almost always enacted in a presentational style.

Examples: In many ways, Dionysus is the first theatrical example of the trickster (see *The Bacchae* by Euripides). The fool as trickster is the precursor to Shakespeare's Puck in *A Midsummer Night's Dream* and to many modern clowns. Examples from classical and later plays include Palaestrio (*The Braggart Warrior* by Plautus), Tony Lumpkin (*She Stoops to Conquer* by O. Goldsmith), Ginifer (*The Knights of the Round Table* by J. Cocteau), The Event (*How I Got That Story* by A. Gray), and Song Lilong (*M. Butterfly* by D. H. Hwang).

17.2. Subtype: Existential Clown

Quality: On the other side of the classical, clever, wisecracking fool is the modern role type that I call the existential clown, trapped within a meaningless universe and joking on the edge of the grave. This type is poetic, unsentimental, nihilistic, minimal, and amoral.

Function: This modern vision of the fool expresses the despair of the clown—an almost logical end to all the humiliations and mockery not only voiced at others, but taken back on oneself. This fool offers no comic relief, but rather points to the absurdity of an existence that is patently foolish. We all live in a fool's paradise, says this fool. The gun that shoots real bullets is as foolish as the one that propels a flag saying "Bang!" This is a complex role type that challenges all viewers to examine the seriousness of their concerns.

Style: The existential clown is enacted in a fully presentational fashion.

Examples: Beckett presents a wide assortment of existential clowns in his minimal plays. An excellent example is Lucky in *Waiting for Godot,* a slave hanging to his master at the end of a rope. The life of this unlucky fool has been reduced to minimal possessions, minimal needs, and minimal actions. His one clownish act is the trick of thinking, which bursts forth in a torrent of words with little rational meaning. His master, Pozzo, is equally clownish, and just as easily is able to reverse roles with Lucky, himself assuming the part of the existential clown.

The Gravedigger in Shakespeare's *Hamlet* is a classical precursor of the modern existential clown. Contemporary examples include Conrad Gerhart (*How the Rent Gets Paid* by J. Weiss) and Willy the Clown (*The Regard of Flight* by B. Irwin).

18. Role Type: Ambivalent One

Quality: This role type is noted by the confused state it foists upon a character. The ambivalent one thinks too much, believing in the validity of two alternative courses of action and thus often unable to act.

Function: The ambivalent one's function is to remain in a state of inaction, a slave to opposing thoughts. Often, when the ambivalent one finally acts, the action has destructive consequences.

Examples: In many ways, Hamlet is the exemplary ambivalent man, described by Shakespeare as "sicklied o'er with the pale cast of thought." Other classical examples include Segismundo (*Life Is a Dream* by P. Calderon) and Wallenstein (*Wallenstein* by F. Schiller). A. Strindberg's Miss Julie in the play of the same name is a strong modern example, as is Joe Bonaparte in *Golden Boy* by C. Odets. In the case of contemporary black theatre, the ambivalent one becomes caught between two cultures as well as two contradictory ways of being. Such characters populate the plays of A. Baraka (e.g., Ray Foote in *The Toilet*) and A. Kennedy (e.g., Sarah the Negro in *Funnyhouse of a Negro*).

18.1. Subtype: Disguised One

Quality: The notion of disguise and mask permeates almost all genres of theatre, as it encapsulates the essence of the dramatic act—the taking on of a persona, the obscuring of the actor in order to reveal the character. As a subtype of the ambivalent one, the disguised one may take on a double identity purposefully, in order to realize a moral objective. Disguise is also evident as one unknowingly takes on a false persona and thus appears foolish. This situation, leading to mistaken identity, becomes a major element in dramatic literature.

Function: There are many dramatic purposes for disguise. Shakespeare presents a variety of women, such as Viola (*Twelfth Night*), Julia (*The Two Gentlemen of Verona*), Rosalind (*As You Like It*), and Helena (*All's Well That Ends Well*), who mask their identities in order to get their men. So, too, do the men employ disguise, but for different purposes: Falstaff (*The Merry Wives of Windsor*), in a dress and horns, to attempt a seduction; Hamlet, in the garb of madman and fool, to dig at the truth by means of assuming a lowly status. The disguise is used as a means to approach the truth or the object of desire indirectly. In a case of mistaken identity, the disguised one is unaware and thus plays the simpleton, opening himself up to ridicule.

Style: The disguised one is generally a presentational character.

Examples: The classical Dionysus (*The Frogs* by Aristophanes) is an early example of a disguised one. Aside from ample Shakespearian examples (see above), others include Christian (*Cyrano de Bergerac* by E. Rostand), Shen Te/Shui Ta (*The Good Woman of Setzuan* by B.

Brecht), Sizwe Banzi (*Sizwe Banzi Is Dead* by A. Fugard), and Superman (*Superman* by R. Benton and D. Newman).

Examples of mistaken identity include Menaechmus of Syracuse (*The Menaechmi* by Plautus), Antipholus of Syracuse (*The Comedy of Errors* by Shakespeare), Dromio of Syracuse (*The Boys from Syracuse* by G. Abbott, R. Rodgers, and L. Hart), and Gregor Samsa (*Metamorphosis,* adaptation of F. Kafka story by C. Dizenzo).

18.2. Subtype: Double

Quality: In modern drama, the unconsciously disguised character takes on a more psychological function, offering the idea of an alter ego or double that reveals a hidden part of the personality. This role type is mysterious, revelatory, probing.

Function: The double functions to reveal a hidden part of the character's personality.

Style: The double is an abstraction and is enacted in a stylized way.

Examples: As this is a modern type, we find examples in such plays as *A Man's a Man* by B. Brecht, where the simple worker, Galy Gay, is transformed into the human fighting machine, Jeraiah Jip. The characters in C. Churchill's *Cloud Nine* confound sexual and political points of view by presenting a double ethnicity (e.g., a black African servant played by a white man), a double sexuality (e.g., men played by women and vice versa), and an open bisexuality within and between the characters. Other examples include Mr. Hyde (*Dr. Jekyll and Mr. Hyde,* adaptation of R. L. Stevenson novel by D. Edgar), Zarathoustra (*Zarathoustra* by J. L. Barrault), and Arlie (*Getting Out* by M. Norman).

19. Role Type: Critic

Quality: Rising above the great unwashed masses, this snobbish type takes on a superior attitude and doles out judgments on all those who fall short of the intellectual or moral standards of the day. The critic is harsh, superior in attitude, punitive, and often self-righteous.

Function: The function of the critic is to assume a superior, lofty attitude and from that perch to pass judgment on a work of art, a person's character, a social or moral issue, or a triviality such as the cut of one's clothes.

Style: Many critics are presented in a farcical style, well fitting the satirical points of view of their creators (e.g., Aristophanes, Sheridan, and Shaw, among many others).

Examples: A late 18th-century play, *The Critic*, by R. Sheridan, introduces the farcical theatre critics Dangle and Sneer, whose names well exemplify their critical facilities. No less of a satirist than G. B. Shaw offers his own version in Flawner Bannal (*Fanny's First Play*). Even in his linguist, Henry Higgins, in *Pygmalion* (and its musical version, *My Fair Lady* by A. J. Lerner and F. Loewe), we find the critic of the social order employing his critical skills to redo the world in his own image. Other examples include Sheridan Whiteside (*The Man Who Came to Dinner* by G. Kaufman and M. Hart) and Moon and Birdboot (*The Real Inspector Hound* by T. Stoppard).

20. Role Type: Wise Person (see also Visionary)

Quality: This type possesses a genuine knowledge and insight concerning a particular issue.

Function: The wise person points out the truth and makes sense of that which is incomprehensible or unclear to others. This role type is in the tradition of the Greek Athena and the Judaic King Solomon.

Examples: In *The Eumenides* by Aeschylus, Athena appears as a judge who will organize a tribunal, then cast the decisive vote that will seal the fate of Orestes. Athena in her wisdom is fully able to resolve this complex case by appeasing the Dionysian Eumenides and diffusing their terrible wrath through offering them a prominent position within Athenian society. As prototype, Athena has spawned endless wise people, including the Elizabethan Helena from Shakespeare's *All's Well That Ends Well*; the 18th-century Sultan Saladin from G. E. Lessing's *Nathan the Wise*; and the modern, earthy Solomon from A. Miller's *The Price*.

20.1. Subtype: Intellectual

Quality: The intellectual is analytical, critical, knowledgeable, and scholarly, though sometimes uninsightful and uncreative. This role type possesses a certain wisdom, but tends to subsist too fully within a cognitive world.

Function: The function of the intellectual is to study and analyze ideas and to understand the workings of systems and processes, sometimes at the expense of a more heartfelt or intuitive knowledge.

Examples: Prospero (*The Tempest* by Shakespeare), Faust (*Faust* by J. W. von Goethe), Lovborg (*Hedda Gabler* by H. Ibsen), The Father (*Six Characters in Search of an Author* by L. Pirandello), Isaac Newton (*In Good King Charles's Golden Days* by G. B. Shaw), Lauffer (*The Tutor,* adaptation of J. Lenz novel by B. Brecht), Jimmy (*Translations* by B. Friel), and Philip (*The Philanthropist* by C. Hampton).

20.2. Subtype: PseudoIntellectual/Pedant

Quality: This type is pretentious, egotistical, foolish, and often arrogant.

Function: The pseudointellectual displays ignorance while attempting to display wisdom.

Style: The pseudointellectual tends to be enacted in a stylized, presentational manner.

Examples: This is a very popular character type who, like other kinds of fools, offers comic relief—in this case, a means for audiences to release their own tendencies toward pretentiousness. Examples throughout theatre history include Socrates (*The Clouds* by Aristophanes), Dottore (various *commedia dell'arte* scripts), Edward Kno'well (*Every Man in His Humour* by B. Jonson), Philaminta (*The Learned Ladies* by Molière), Mr. Sparkish (*The Country Wife* by W. Wycherley), Puff (*The Critic* by R. Sheridan), Serebriakoff (*Uncle Vanya* by A. Chekhov), The Old Man (*The Chairs* by E. Ionesco), and George (*Jumpers* by T. Stoppard).

DOMAIN: AFFECTIVE

Classification: MORAL

21. Role Type: Innocent (see also Child and Beauty)

Quality: In quality, the innocent is pure, moral, and chaste, unself-conscious and intending no harm or humiliation toward another. The innocent, as a foil for the tyrant and deceiver, is a moral figure—a reminder of the gentler, purer virtues that reside within the human heart.

Function: The function of the innocent is to remain pure and unspoiled, committed to the virtues of chastity and loyalty, even in the face of a repressive and threatening authority.

Style: The style of the innocent is presentational, as this is an idealized role, familiar in myth, fable, and fairy tale. Even as theatrical forms have become more representational, the innocent role type has subsisted as a reminder of the primal, universal struggle between the forces of darkness and light.

Examples: One example of the innocent in Renaissance theatre

is the plain-speaking and loyal Cordelia in Shakespeare's *King Lear.*
The role type of the innocent has subsisted in endless sacred and pro-
fane characters as far apart as Joan of Arc (see for example *The Maid
of Orleans* by F. Schiller) and Billy Budd (in the play of the same name,
adaptation of H. Melville story by L. Coxe and R. Chapman). Other
examples include Hippolytus (*Hippolytus* by Euripides), Issac (*Abraham and Isaac* by Anonymous), Justina (*The Wonder-Working Magician* by P. Calderon), Agnes (*The School for Wives* by Molière), Consuelo
(*He Who Gets Slapped* by L. Andreyev), Josie (*A Moon for the Misbegotten* by E. O'Neill), Kilroy (*Camino Real* by T. Williams), Teresa (*The
Hostage* by B. Behan), and Agnes (*Agnes of God* by J. Pielmeir).

22. Role Type: Villain

Quality: The villain takes a moral position opposite to that of
the hero. He wants, in either a material or moral sense, that which
the hero has (e.g., power, wealth, status, righteousness). In quality,
villains may be ignorant and brutish, but more often, especially when
well developed, they reveal a certain Machiavellian wisdom that
matches the hero's more righteous or innocent wisdom. As heroes
tend to be moral characters, villains tend to be either immoral or
(when complexly drawn) amoral.

Function: The villain's purpose is generally to struggle with the
heroes and to attempt to wrest power from them, often using underhanded means.

Style: Generally speaking, the more sophisticated the villain in
terms of intelligence, awareness, and power, the greater the opportun-
ities for a psychologically realistic performance. Such a complex villain like Shakespeare's Iago in *Othello*, although written with a high
degree of style, can be portrayed in a more modern representational
form. Unlike some of Shakespeare's other villains, such as Edmund,
Regan, and Goneril in *King Lear,* Iago is a person of complex motivation who functions not only to satisfy his need for revenge at being
denied an expected promotion, but also to gratify his lust for power,
control, and ultimately destruction.

Examples: Other villains include Creon (*Antigone* and *Oedipus
at Colonus* by Sophocles), Flamineo (*The White Devil* by J. Webster),
Regina Giddens (*The Little Foxes* by L. Hellman), Salieri (*Amadeus* by
P. Shaffer), and Paul (*Six Degrees of Separation* by J. Guare).

23. Role Type: The Deceiver (see also Beast, Immoralist, and Demon)

Quality: Villainous characters and others, such as hypocrites,
charlatans, impostors, thieves, traitors, and con artists, belong to a

more generic type that can be called the deceiver. The deceiver is treacherous, underhanded, and immoral; a foil for the hero and innocent; and often a pariah.

Function: All deceivers serve a general function within drama—to lead the heroes and others astray, thus promoting their own self-interest. Some are not content unless they engineer a large-scale catastrophe. Others, less bloodthirsty, are satisfied with the deception itself, and more concerned with their own personal gain than with the punishment of others whom they perceive as threats. Deceivers function as antagonists and thus have proven indispensable throughout the history of drama. Sometimes charming, like Fagin in the musical *Oliver!* (adaptation of C. Dickens novel by L. Bart), and sometimes brutal, like the Hitler parody, Arturo Ui in *The Resistible Rise of Arturo Ui*, by B. Brecht, these characters never cease to engage audiences needing to exorcise their own subversive tendencies.

Style: See 22 above.

Examples: The examples cited in 22 above apply equally to this role type. Further examples, encompassing hypocrites, charlatans, con artists, and thieves, include Pisthetaurus (*The Birds* by Aristophanes), Subtle, Face, and Doll Common (*The Alchemist* by B. Jonson), Maskwell (*The Double Dealer* by W. Congreve), Klestakhov (*The Inspector General* by N. Gogol), and Roma (*Glengarry Glen Ross* by D. Mamet).

24. Role Type: Moralist (see also Innocent)

Quality: This type is highly moralistic, pious, chaste, and self-righteous, seeing most issues as either good or bad, with few shades in between.

Function: The moralist takes an extreme position, asserting and protecting a highly valued ideal, principle or belief.

Examples: Good Deeds (*Everyman* by Anonymous), Isabella (*Measure for Measure* by Shakespeare), Samson (*Samson Agonistes* by J. Milton), Adam Trueman (*Fashion* by A. C. Mowatt), Anton (*Maria Magdalena* by F. Hebbel), John Brown (*John Brown's Body* by S. V. Benet), John Proctor (*The Crucible* by A. Miller).

24.1. Subtype: Hypocritical Moralist

Quality: The ancient Greek New Comedy introduced a character type that appears to be highly pious, yet proves to be a hypocrite. This alternative type is immoral, using the moralist role as a mask to exploit others.

Function: The hypocritical moralist dons the mask of piety in order to satisfy personal ambitions.

Style: This type is generally enacted in a presentational style.

Examples: We find an early example of the hypocritical moralist in Menander's *The Arbitration,* where the seemingly virtuous Charisius marries the daughter of a wealthy businessman, and is soon exposed as a womanizer and carouser. The hypocritical moralist has become a popular figure in the hands of various comic playwrights. One of its most famous exemplars, Molière's Tartuffe in the play of the same name, plays this role in order to achieve power over those with more goods but less wit. Tartuffe has inspired translators, actors, directors, and audiences for some 300 years. One reason might be that the hypocrite calls forth the two contradictory human pulls toward altruism and egotism, pointing to the delicate balance between social responsibility and exploitation. Further examples include Rabbi Zeal-of-the-Land Busy (*Bartholomew Fair* by B. Jonson), Robespierre (*Danton's Death* by G. Büchner), Judge Adam (*The Broken Jug* by H. von Kleist), and Miss Gilchrist (*The Hostage* by B. Behan).

24.2. Subtype: Idealist

Quality: This is a romantic type, fiercely committed to a principle or ideology.

Function: Idealists remain true to a given ideal or ideology that provides meaning to their lives.

Examples: Examples include Antigone (*Antigone* by Sophocles), Brutus (*Julius Caesar* by Shakespeare), Dr. Stockmann (*An Enemy of the People* by H. Ibsen), Edmund (*Long Day's Journey into Night* by E. O'Neill), Don Quixote (*Camino Real* by T. Williams), Arthur (*Tango* by S. Mrozek), and Sidney Brustein (*The Sign in Sidney Brustein's Window* by L. Hansberry).

25. Role Type: Immoralist

Quality: This type, which includes rogue, lecher, courtesan/prostitute, and pimp, is earthy, licentious, lusty, unconventional, and immoral. Some are forced into the role by economic circumstances and/or social oppression.

Function: Immoralists satisfy their lust at the expense of others and act outside the confines of the law. The oppressed immoralist attempts to survive hardship by taking on a criminal persona.

Examples: The prostitute has the distinction of being not only the oldest profession, but also one of the most often repeated dramatic types. Erotium, the courtesan in *The Menaechmi* by Plautus, foreshadows endless low comedic illustrations of the lusty bawd. This role type also includes the pimp, represented by Plautus's Cappadox in *Curculio*. Other examples of immoralists include Mistress Overdone (*Measure for Measure* by Shakespeare), Marie (*Woyzeck* by G. Büchner), Mr. Dudley Smooth (*Money* by E. Bulwer-Lytton), Anna Christie (*Anna Christie* by E. O'Neill), Carmen, Executioner, Judge, and Irma (*The Balcony* by J. Genet), Jenny (*The Threepenny Opera* by B. Brecht and K. Weill), Kitty (*The Time of Your Life* by W. Saroyan), Senex (*A Funny Thing Happened on the Way to the Forum* by B. Shevelove, L. Gilbert, and S. Sondheim), and The Engineer (*Miss Saigon* by A. Boublil, C.-M. Schonberg, and R. Maltby).

25.1. Subtype: Libertine

Quality: The libertine is uninhibited, pleasure-seeking, charming, seductive, and often childlike.

Function: This type seeks pleasure, usually though not necessarily at the expense of others.

Examples: Philolaches (*The Haunted House* by Plautus), Titania (*A Midsummer Night's Dream* by Shakespeare), Don Juan (*The Trickster of Seville and His Guest of Stone* by T. de Molina), Dorimant (*The Man of Mode* by G. Etherege), Lulu (*Pandora's Box* by F. Wedekind), Macheath (*The Threepenny Opera* by B. Brecht and K. Weill), The Marquis de Sade (*Marat/Sade* by P. Weiss), and Sally Bowles (*I Am a Camera* by J. Van Druten and *Cabaret* by J. Masteroff, J. Kander, and F. Ebb).

25.2. Subtype: Adulterer/Adulteress

Quality: The adulterer/adulteress is a restless hedonist, often sneaky and bored, in search of a new sexual conquest.

Function: The function of this type is to satisfy a need for sex and adventure, and to alleviate for a time a sense of boredom.

Examples: Adultery, real and imagined, plays a large part in Roman comedy. One of the most enduring examples appears in Plautus's *Amphitryon*. The adulterer is a god, Jupiter, who cuckolds Amphitryon by assuming his shape and seducing his wife. And so begins a long tradition of adulterous seduction and complicity, culminating in at least 38 Amphitryon plays alone (see J. Giraudoux's *Amphitryon 38*). Other examples include Wife (*Johan, Johan* by J. Heywood), Mistress Arden (*Arden of Feversham* by Anonymous), John Middleton (*The Constant Wife* by W. S. Maugham), Stella (*The Magnificent Cuckold* by F. Crommelynck), Jerry and Emma (*Betrayal* by H. Pinter), and Merteuil (*Les Liaisons Dangereuses*, adaptation of C. de Laclos novel by C. Hampton).

26. Role Type: Victim

Quality: The victim, in its several forms of scapegoat, hostage, prisoner, and slave, is vulnerable, trapped, defenseless, under the control of another's will or the will of fate. Many of the Greek heroic figures begin as victims but are ultimately powerful enough to battle against their victimizers. Many of the antiheroic victims in later plays do not prove as powerful and remain forever entrenched in their oppressive conditions.

Function: The function of the victim is to succumb, to give up control.

Examples: The role of victim in many ways springs from the Greek notion of tragic hero. Tragic heroes go on a search because they have been victimized in some significant way. Oedipus, Orestes, Electra, Iphigenia, and Prometheus are all initially victims. They are victimized by the gods, as in the case of Prometheus; by oppressive authorities, as in the case of Antigone; by embedded family antagonisms, as in the case of Orestes and Electra; by fathers, as in the case of Iphigenia; and by the classical victimizers, fate and pride, as in the case of Oedipus. To the extent that they do battle with the forces that victimize them, they achieve the status of tragic hero. Less heroic victims include Desdemona (*Othello* by Shakespeare), Phaedra (*Phaedra* by J. Racine), Leslie (*The Hostage* by B. Behan), The Dark Man (*The Woman* by E. Bond), Craig Donner (*The Normal Heart* by L. Kramer), and Slaves (*Slaveship* by A. Baraka).

26.1. Subtype: Martyr

Quality: This type of victim chooses self-sacrifice in the service of a specific cause or ideal. The martyr is principled and often dogmatic.

Function: Martyrs commit themselves fully and utterly to a cause; they rescue others from a painful existence, and in doing so sacrifice their own needs.

Examples: Prometheus (*Prometheus Bound* by Aeschylus) can be seen as the prototypical classical martyr, who stoically bears his torturous existence in the service of bringing fire and light to humankind. And at the heels of Prometheus is the prototypical Christian martyr, Jesus Christ (see *The Passion Play* by Anonymous and *Jesus Christ Superstar* by T. Rice and A. Lloyd Webber), who embodies the further purpose of taking on a painful existence so that others might be liberated from their pain. Other examples include Joan of Arc (*Joan of Arc* by P. MacKaye), Archbishop Thomas Becket of Canterbury

(*Murder in the Cathedral* by T. S. Eliot), and Larry Foreman (*The Cradle Will Rock* by M. Blitzstein).

26.2. Subtype: Self-Serving Martyr

Quality: An alternative type of martyr feigns self-sacrifice and is manipulative, self-involved, and self-pitying.

Function: This type procures sympathy and instills guilt, manipulating others in order to to get his/her way.

Examples: Although this type is well known in popular fiction and the mass media as "the Jewish mother," its prototype is in the character of Falstaff (see especially *Henry IV, Part II* by Shakespeare). Contemporary examples include Felix (*The Odd Couple* by N. Simon), Mrs. Beckoff (*Torch Song Trilogy* H. Fierstein), and Allan Felix (*Play It Again, Sam* by W. Allen).

27. Role Type: Opportunist

Quality: The opportunist and its relation, the demagogue, is referred to by Arrowsmith (1970) as "a politician without a policy" (p. 10). This type is characterized by unscrupulousness, willfulness, cunning, and a restless energy that is not easily satisfied. Such a role type is motivated by the acquisition of power and status for its own sake.

Function: The dramatic function of the opportunist is to accumulate that power and status, without concern for those whose power is diminished in the quest.

Examples: In *The Birds* by Aristophanes, we meet the Athenian Pisthetairos, a deceptively simple character who, along with his companion, Euelpides, turns his back on the abuses of the city to seek a simple Utopia among the birds. In fact, Pisthetairos manages to manipulate the birds in such a way that he is able to realize a personal goal of power and control. The Utopian dreamer thus becomes entrepreneur, politician, and imperialist, conquering the beings of the sky—both the birds and the gods—through cunning and power. The role of the opportunist often appears darkly in the shapes of politicians, like Shakespeare's Richard III; tyrants, like Brecht's Arturo Ui; and businessmen, like Joe Keller in A. Miller's *All My Sons*. Other examples include Lady Macbeth (*Macbeth* by Shakespeare), Macbird (*Macbird* by B. Garson), Engstrand (*Ghosts* by H. Ibsen), Klestakhov (*The Inspector General* by N. Gogol), Eddie (*Tango* by S. Mrozek), Lambert LaRoux (*Pravda* by H. Brenton and D. Hare), and Levene (*Glengarry Glen Ross* by D. Mamet).

28. Role Type: Bigot

Quality: The bigot, inclusive of qualities shared by racists, sexists, misogynists, and misanthropes, is intolerant, self-righteous, chauvinistic, and angry.

Function: The bigot functions to scapegoat, harass, offend, incite and provoke others. This type has proliferated in drama when racial, sexual, or national tensions are high within a particular culture.

Style: In style, this type often appears overblown and overstated to make a political point about the nature of bigotry.

Examples: The role type is to be found often in contemporary forms of street theatre. For example, The Bread and Puppet Theatre employs a large, bulbous puppet called Uncle Fatso and an overblown, top-hatted Uncle Sam to represent such ills as greed and imperialism. On the other hand, the role of bigot is played more realistically within such modern dramas as *A Streetcar Named Desire* by T. Williams, which reveals the effects of Stanley Kowalski's bigoted behavior upon two sisters. Other examples include Cnemon (*Dyskolos* by Menander), Petruchio (*The Taming of the Shrew* by Shakespeare), Alceste (*The Misanthrope* by Molière), Parris (*The Crucible* by A. Miller), Hally ("*Master Harold*". . . *and the Boys* by A. Fugard), and Governor Lester What's-His-Name (*Red, White and Maddox* by D. Tucker).

29. Role Type: Avenger

Quality: The avenger is a role type that is marked by an obsessive need for revenge. Avengers are often ruthless in their passion for settling a score, living by the credo "An eye for an eye and a tooth for a tooth."

Function: The function of the avenger is to redress a perceived grievance through an act of revenge, which in drama is often a violent act. The avenger well encapsulates the rage of audience members, who, with few socially acceptable places to vent their rage, may need revenge plays to vicariously avenge a wrong in their own lives.

Examples: The Western tradition of revenge plays begins with the Greeks. The powerful characters of Medea (*Medea* by Euripedes) and Ajax (*Ajax* by Sophicles) are both motivated by revenge; the former commits a brutal act of infanticide and the latter an act of suicide in the heat of rage. The most celebrated cycle of revenge plays is Aeschylus's *Orestia*, which continues the revenge motif within the House of Atreus by pitting the avenger Clytemnestra against her husband, Agamemnon; and their children, Orestes and Electra, against their murderous mother. These remarkable characters reappear in many forms throughout Western drama, most notably in Jacobean revenge tragedies. Such moderns as J.-P. Sartre and E. O'Neill have used the characters from the *Orestia* to make their dark critiques of modern existence in *The Flies* and *Mourning Becomes Electra*, respectively. Other examples include Atreus (*Thyestes* by Seneca), Vendice (*The Revenger's Tragedy* by C. Tourneur), Evadne (*The Maid's Tragedy* by F. Beaumont and J. Fletcher), Revenge (*The Spanish Tragedy* by T. Kyd), Clair Zachanassia (*The Visit* by F. Dürrenmatt), and Marjorie (*Extremities* by W. Mastrosimone).

30. Role Type: Helper

Quality: The helper is moral, unselfish, supportive, and altruistic. This type also appears as the good friend and the good Samaritan.

Function: The helper functions to move the hero or protagonist further along his path or to rescue another from difficult circumstances, remaining loyal throughout the many twists and turns of the journey.

Examples: Shakespeare's *King Lear* is a powerful play about deception and cruelty. Yet embedded within the nightmarish universe of Lear and Gloucester are the noble and loyal daughter and son, Cordelia and Edgar. Lear's loyal vassal, Kent, is a prototypical helper who endures humiliation and death threats in order to insure the safety of his master, however foolish that master has become. The helper certainly has precedents in Greek drama, most notably in the devotion and help offered by Antigone to both her father and brother. So, too, does this role type extend throughout dramatic literature, providing many Hamlets with their Horatios, many Blanche DuBois with their Stellas. Other examples include: Hermes (*The Eumenides* by Aeschylus), Trueman (*The London Merchant* by G. Lillo), Fidelia (*The Plain Dealer* by W. Wycherley), Curt (*The Dance of Death* by A. Strindberg), Amanda Smith (*No Time for Comedy* by S. N. Behrman), Sagredo (*Galileo* by B. Brecht), and Mame (*Auntie Mame* by J. Lawrence and R. Lee).

31. Role Type: Philistine

Quality: This type includes boors, idlers, and gossips, those who talk too much with too little imagination. These philistines are unrefined, common, conventional, boorish, smug, one-dimensional, and pretentious.

Function: The philistine provides comic relief and satire, and warns audiences not to take themselves and their judgments too seriously.

Style: Generally broad and farcical, the philistine has taken on more complexity in the modern drama.

Examples: These characters abound in such Molière farces as *The Learned Ladies, The Misanthrope,* and *The Would-Be Gentleman.* They proliferate in British Restoration comedy and modern drama. Examples include Malvolio (*Twelfth Night* by Shakespeare), Sir John Brute (*The Provok'd Wife* by J. Vanbrugh), Ivan Prisypkin (*The Bedbug* by V. Mayakovsky), and Wilma and Martha (*The Rimers of Eldritch* by L. Wilson).

32. Role Type: Miser

Quality: The miser is tight and controlling, power-hungry, obsessional with material things, and possessive with human beings.

Function: The miser functions to hoard things of perceived value. His greedy actions come with a price tag, however. For his tightness, he is repaid by the pain of separation from intimacy, like King Midas, whose touch turns his loved ones to gold.

Examples: Plautus offers an early version of the miser in his play *The Pot of Gold.* The character, Euclio, broadly drawn, is described in the play as follows: "when he goes to sleep, he'll tie the bellows around his throat . . . lest he should waste his breath." He becomes the prototype for such dramatists as Molière and O'Neill, whose Harpagon (*The Miser*) and James Tyrone (*Long Day's Journey into Night*) well exemplify the tight and controlling qualities of the miser.

33. Role Type: Coward

Quality: This is an unheroic type, fearful and easily threatened, unwilling to take risks.

Function: The function of the coward is to succumb to fear and shrink from confronting dangerous and challenging situations.

Examples: Parolles (*All's Well That Ends Well* by Shakespeare), Sir Andrew Aguecheek (*Twelfth Night* by Shakespeare), Ubu (*Ubu Roi* by A. Jarry), Garcin (*No Exit* by J.-P. Sartre), and Don (*American Buffalo* by D. Mamet).

33.1. Subtype: Braggart/Braggart Warrior (see also Narcissist)

Quality: This type is one who knows too little but says too much. In quality, the braggart is ignorant, brash, foolish, self-righteous, and pretentious—all form with little substance. The braggart warrior extols his virtues both on the battlefield and in the boudoir, but, when challenged, falls short in both arenas.

Function: The braggart's aggressive brashness functions to mask the character's basic sense of inferiority. Through comic catharsis, the audience releases its own sense of inadequacy when participating in that of the broadly drawn boaster.

Style: The style of the braggart role tends to be that of low comedy—slapstick, burlesque, farce. In the Italian *commedia dell'arte,* the braggart becomes the mock-heroic Capitano, a man of many medals but little mettle.

Examples: In Plautus's *Miles Gloriosus,* we find the prototype for the braggart. Plautus's Pyrgopolynices attempts to prove his sexual prowess by capturing a young courtesan, but is tricked into relinquishing his would-be mistress by a clever slave. In the end, he is exposed as an adulterer and punished. At one point, he exclaims that his descendants will endure "for a thousand years, from one age to the next." This stock character has indeed endured, spawning such creations as N. Udall's Ralph Roister Doister in the play of the same name, Jonson's Captain Bobadill (*Every Man in His Humour*), P. Corneille's Matamore (*The Comic Illusion*), G. Büchner's The Drum Major (*Woyzeck*), and the endearing Cowardly Lion (*The Wizard of Oz,* by L. F. Baum).

34. Role Type: Parasite

Quality: This type is by nature a hanger-on, a flatterer, a leech and fawner, one who sponges off others in order to increase his own status.

Function: The parasite functions to increase his own fortunes by attaching himself to one of a perceived higher status.

Style: Although many audience members find this type repulsive, it is often presented with enough style to allow viewers to laugh at their own proclivities toward sponging.

Examples: Plautus's *The Menaechmi,* a play of mistaken identity that became the model for both Shakespeare's *The Comedy of Errors,* and the modern musical *The Boys from Syracuse* by G. Abbott, R. Rodgers, and L. Hart, offers a number of stock comedic characters, among them Peniculus or "Sponge," the parasite. The Sponge as a type is abundant in Elizabethan theatre, a prominent example being Mosca ("The Fly"), who sucks up to all, including his master, Volpone ("The Fox"), for his own gain (*Volpone* by B. Jonson). Volpone and Mosca have been born again in an opera, *Volpone* by F. Burt, and a musical comedy, *The Sly Fox* by L. Gelbart. Modern drama presents its own parade of parasites, well exemplified by Mrs. Shin in Brecht's *The Good Woman of Setzuan,* who suddenly cozies up to Shen Te, the generous but penniless prostitute, once she has been bequeathed a small fortune by the gods. Other examples include Gnatho (*The Eunuch* by Terence), Merygreek (*Ralph Roister Doister* by N. Udall), and Charlie Fox (*Speed-the-Plow* by D. Mamet).

35. Role Type: Survivor

Quality: The survivor, persistent in the face of threat, is morally courageous, tough, and resilient.

Function: The function of the survivor is to endure and exhibit moral courage in the face of often overwhelming obstacles.

Examples: Brecht's most famous survivor, Mother Courage (*Mother Courage and Her Children*), does whatever she must to protect herself and those close to her. The survivor role is, with some notable exceptions, a modern one. One could argue that the classical tragic heroes have qualities of the survivor, in that they struggle against an array of external antagonists and internal demons. Yet most do not survive. Unwilling to compromise a moral position, Oedipus puts out his eyes, Antigone is led to her death, Lear goes mad, and Hamlet falls victim to his own revenge. This is not so with Mother Courage; in a contradictory or amoral universe, she behaves amorally. Further examples throughout theatre history include Hecuba (*The Trojan Women* by Euripides), Pericles (*Pericles* by Shakespeare), Andromache (*Andromache* by J. Racine), Frau Wolff (*The Beaver Coat* by G. Hauptmann), Sonya (*Uncle Vanya* by A. Chekhov), Galileo (*Galileo* by B. Brecht), Jacobowsky (*Jacobowsky and the Colonel* by F. Werfel), Juno (*Juno and the Paycock* by S. O'Casey), Anne Frank (*The Diary of Anne Frank* by F. Goodrich and A. Hackett), Lena Younger (*A Raisin in the Sun* by L. Hansberry), and John Kani and Winston Ntshona (*The Island* by A. Fugard, J. Kani, and W. Ntshona).

Classification: FEELING STATES

36. Role Type: Zombie

Quality: The zombie, a type of living dead, is emotionally frozen, lifeless, amoral.

Function: This modern type functions to shut down all feeling in order to protect oneself from memory and intimacy.

Style: The zombie is, for the most part, enacted in a presentational manner.

Examples: Robots (*R. U. R.* by K. Capek), Peter (*The Zoo Story* by E. Albee), Charlotte Corday (*Marat/Sade* by P. Weiss), Joe Egg (*A Day in the Death of Joe Egg* by P. Nichols), Emily Stilsm (*Wings* by A. Kopit), Bam, Bom, Bim, Bem, and Voice of Bam (*What Where* by S. Beckett), Ensemble (*The Dead Class* by T. Kantor), and Deborah (*A Kind of Alaska* by H. Pinter).

36.1. Subtype: Lost One (see also Pariah)

Quality: The lost one is estranged and alienated, amoral, lacking a sense of purpose or understanding of his/her's place in the universe.

Function: This type accepts meaninglessness as a given and, despite occasional bewilderment, endures without questioning the purpose of life.

Examples: The many lost characters who appear in Chekhov's plays are estranged and alienated from both their societies and inner lives. These are people who once had wealth and status, youth and dreams, but now spend their time trying to live with the consequences of their loss. This modern character is well exemplified in the once powerful and glamorous Madame Ranevskaya (*The Cherry Orchard*), about to lose her beloved cherry orchard, the final symbol of status and joy. Many of the modern lost ones appear in much darker, depressive tones than Chekhov's characters, who live with their quiet desperation in an almost clownish fashion. As early as 1836, G. Büchner presented an example of the lost one in Woyzeck (*Woyzeck*), a nonentity struggling against indifference and betrayal in the world outside and inside. A plethora of lost ones has appeared prominently in the 20th century as a response to the general existential condition most clearly articulated by Camus in his novel *The Stranger* (1942/1988). In the modern theatre we find such lost ones as O'Neill's beast-like Yank Smith (*The Hairy Ape*), P. Lagerkvist's (*The Man Without a Soul*), and Beckett's insulated Krapp (*Krapp's Last Tape*), a waste product of the modern age. In the extreme, the Beckett lost one becomes a zombie, emotionally frozen and lifeless, needing desperately to shut down all feeling in order to protect himself from memory and intimacy. The lost one accepts the silence or death of God as a given. Some, like Madame Ranevskaya and Krapp, endure. Others, from the darker world of Woyzeck and Yank Smith, either commit suicide or are callously murdered. Further examples include The Stranger (*To Damascus, Part I* by A. Strindberg), Corporal Beckmann (*The Man Outside* by W. Borchert), and Edgar Valpor (*The Water Hen* by S. Witkiewicz).

37. Role Type: Malcontent

Quality: Malcontents are pessimistic, unhappy creatures who can not seem to live comfortably within the established order.

Function: Malcontents react negatively to the perceived injustices of the established order. They shake things up and force others to respond to their open critiques of the norm.

Examples: Orestes (*The Libation Bearers* by Aeschylus), Macbeth (*Macbeth* by Shakespeare), Hedda Gabler (*Hedda Gabler* by H. Ibsen), Sonya and Uncle Vanya (*Uncle Vanya* by A. Chekhov), Olga, Masha, and Irina (*The Three Sisters* by A. Chekhov), Julie (*Miss Julie* by A. Strindberg), and Sweeney Todd (*Sweeney Todd* by H. Wheeler and S. Sondheim).

37.1. Subtype: Cynic

Quality: This type of malcontent is sardonic, critical, intellectual, pessimistic, and cold.

Function: The cynic attempts to prove that life is futile and to maintain power by defending against feeling.

Examples: Brighella (various *commedia dell'arte* scripts), Apemantus (*Timon of Athens* by Shakespeare), Frate Timoteo (*Mandragola* by N. Machiavelli), Dr. Relling (*The Wild Duck* by H. Ibsen), Judge Brack (*Hedda Gabler* by H. Ibsen), Belcredi (*Henry IV* by L. Pirandello), James Tyrone, Jr. (*A Moon for the Misbegotten* by E. O'Neill), Ben Butley (*Butley* by S. Gray), and Brecht (*Tales from Hollywood* by C. Hampton).

37.2. Subtype: Hothead

Quality: Whereas the cynic is intellectual, the hothead is emotional, impulsive, irrational, given to violent outbursts.

Function: The hothead expresses hurt, anger, and rage openly and directly.

Examples: Medea (*Medea* by Euripides), Hotspur (*Henry IV, Part I* by Shakespeare), Goneril (*King Lear* by Shakespeare), Tybalt (*Romeo and Juliet* by Shakespeare), Jimmy Porter (*Look Back in Anger* by J. Osborne), and Levee (*Ma Rainey's Black Bottom* by A. Wilson).

37.3. Subtype: Shrew

Quality: The shrew is angry, strident, nagging, and annoying.

Function: Shrews express themselves in a harsh, strident manner in order to feel powerful and attain a desired goal.

Example: The Wife (*The Menaechmi* by Plautus), Kate (*The Taming of the Shrew* by Shakespeare), Shoemaker's Wife (*The Shoemaker's Prodigious Wife* by F. Garcia Lorca), Cléante (*Amphitryon* by Molière), Frau Marthe Rull (*The Broken Jug* by H. von Kleist), Megaera (*Androcles and the Lion* by G. B. Shaw), and Agnes (*A Delicate Balance* by E. Albee).

37.4. Subtype: Rebel

Quality: The rebel is discontented with and rejects the established order. This type wages rebellion through war or wit.

Function: Rebels proclaim their discontent through taking action against an established authority. As they assert their acerbic influence throughout the ages, they provide audiences the opportunity to release some of their own anger.

Examples: Lysistrata in the Aristophanes play of the same name represents a clever version of the rebel, as she makes a forceful anti-war statement by encouraging the women of Athens to deny sex to their husbands unless they refrain from waging war. Other witty and/or aggressive rebels throughout theatre history include Cassius (*Julius Caesar* by Shakespeare), William Tell (*William Tell* by F. Schiller), Lieutenant Maryk (*The Caine Mutiny Court-Martial* by H. Wouk), The Living Theatre Ensemble (*Paradise Now* by J. Beck, J. Malina, and ensemble), and McMurphy (*One Flew over the Cuckoo's Nest,* adaptation of K. Kesey novel by D. Wasserman).

38. Role Type: Lover

Quality: As a role type, the lover is romantic and tender, devoted to a mate body and soul.

Function: The lover expresses romantic and passionate feelings toward a love object.

Style: Romantic by nature, the lover tends to be enacted in a stylized fashion, although traditions of psychological realism call for more representational performances.

Examples: Shakespeare's lovers are legion, the most influential being Romeo and Juliet. Here are the star-crossed lovers made more romantic by virtue of the antagonistic and violent society in which they live. In the tradition of *Romeo and Juliet,* we find the popular musical *West Side Story* by A. Laurents, S. Sondheim, and L. Bernstein. A mainstay of theatre, the lover is also exemplified by the following: Pamphilus (*The Woman of Andros* by Terence), Ferdinand and Miranda (*The Tempest* by Shakespeare), Mirabell and Millamant (*The Way* *of the World* by W. Congreve), Elizabeth Barrett and Robert Browning (*The Barretts of Wimpole Street* by R. Besier), George Gibbs and Emily Webb (*Our Town* by T. Wilder), and Tony and Tina (*Tony and Tina's Wedding,* a presentation by Artificial Intelligence).

38.1. Subtype: Narcissist/Egotist (see also Braggart)

Quality: This version of the lover is a person in love with oneself. The narcissist, obsessed with externals and images, is self-involved to the point of being unable to recognize the emotional needs of another.

Function: Narcissists dote upon themselves to such an extent that they effectively shut out intimate relationships with others. They live a life of appearances, of form with little substance.

Examples: Malvolio (*Twelfth Night* by Shakespeare), Cleopatra (*Antony and Cleopatra* by Shakespeare), Henry Higgins (*Pygmalion* by G. B. Shaw), Aubrey Piper (*The Show-Off* by G. Kelly), Jack Boyle (*Juno and the Paycock* by S. O'Casey), Sheridan Whiteside (*The Man Who Came to Dinner* by G. Kaufman and M. Hart), and Eva Peron (*Evita* by T. Rice and A. Lloyd Webber).

39. Role Type: Ecstatic One (see also Dionysian God/Goddess)

Quality: This type appears to be living within an altered state of consciousness. A true Dionysian, this type is transcendent, amoral, possessed, and irrational.

Function: The ecstatic one expresses the irrational, transcendent part of the human psyche and seeks out moments of orgiastic experience.

Style: This type is enacted in a primal, stylized fashion, appealing to the senses and emotions.

Examples: The prototypical ecstatic one is Dionysus, who in many ways presents one of two basic character models for tragic drama (the other being Apollo; see Nietzsche, 1872/1956). Dionysus in person and spirit appears throughout theatre history, and is represented in the classic *The Bacchae* by Euripides and the contemporary *Dionysus in 69* by The Performance Group. Other examples of ecstatic characters are The Furies (*Thyestes* by Seneca), Penthesilea and the Amazons (*Penthesilea* by H. von Kleist), Leah (*The Dybbuk* by S. Ansky), The Flies (*The Flies* by J.-P. Sartre), Dracula and Lucy (*Dracula: Sabbat* by L. Katz), and Rose (*Dancing at Lughnasa* by B. Friel).

CHAPTER TEN

The Taxonomy:
Social Domain

DOMAIN: SOCIAL

Classification: FAMILY

40. Role Type: Mother

Quality: The conventional mother is moral, loving, caring, and nurturing. She is a survivor.

Function: The most basic function of the mother is to protect and nurture her children.

Style: Although sometimes presented in a stylized fashion, like Brecht's Mother Courage, the mother is generally enacted representationally.

Examples: Examples of this "good" mother include Andromache (*The Trojan Women* by Euripides), Constance (*King John* by Shakespeare), Grusha (*The Caucasian Chalk Circle* by B. Brecht), Mama (*I Remember Mama* by J. Van Druten), Linda Loman (*Death of a Salesman* by A. Miller), Thelma (*'Night, Mother* by M. Norman), and Ma Joad (*The Grapes of Wrath,* adaptation of J. Steinbeck novel by F. Galati).

40.1. Subtype: Murderous Mother

Quality: This type of "bad" mother is vengeful, amoral, violent, and murderous.

Function: This mother asserts the Dionysian power of women, which is ecstatic and irrational. She aims to destroy her children.

Style: This dark version of the mother is presented in a stylized, often mythic fashion.

Examples: Medea (*Medea* by Euripides), Agave (*The Bacchae* by Euripides), Athaliah (*Athaliah* by J. Racine), The Mother (*Blood Wedding* by F. Garcia Lorca), Matryona (*The Power of Darkness* by L. Tolstoy), Natella Abashwili (*The Caucasian Chalk Circle* by B. Brecht), and The Mother (*The Screens* by J. Genet).

40.2. Subtype: Revolutionary Mother

Quality: A third version of the mother portrayed in theatre is that of the progressive or revolutionary.

Function: This mother envisions a new moral and political order and fights for its realization. She turns her nurturing instincts toward political as well as personal goals, although sometimes the latter are sacrificed for the former.

Style: The mother as revolutionary is generally portrayed within the sytle of epic or political theatre. However, the human side of this type is also underlined in certain contemporary productions.

Examples: Examples of this type are found in modern and contemporary political and feminist theatre, and include Pelagez Vlassova (*The Mother* by B. Brecht), Sarah (*Chicken Soup with Barley by A. Wesker),* Mollie *(*Mollie Bailey's Traveling Family Circus by M. Terry), and Mother Jones (*Furies of Mother Jones* by M. Klein).

41. Role Type: Wife

Quality: The conventional version of the wife portrayed, with some notable exceptions, throughout much of theatre history is that of the faithful, loving, and caring helper.

Function: This wife's primary function is to take care of husband and home.

Examples: Alcestis (*Alcestis* by Euripides), Desdemona (*Othello* by Shakespeare), Elmire (*Tartuffe* by Molière), Yelena (*Uncle Vanya* by A. Chekhov), Birdie Hubbard (*The Little Foxes* by L. Hellman), Mrs. Antrobus (*The Skin of Our Teeth* by T. Wilder), and Stella (*A Streetcar Named Desire* by T. Williams).

41.1. Subtype: Liberated Wife

Quality: One exception to the norm is the wife who is liberated from a conventional relationship to her husband or struggling to be so.

Function: This alternative wife, in her most fully developed dramatic form, challenges the status quo—first on an internal psychological level, battling her own internal demons of conventionality and passivity; and then on a social level, rebelling against the external forces of oppression, whether her husband or society.

Examples: Although the liberated wife is a modern convention, she has appeared in earlier plays. She is found in Greek comedy in the character of Myrrhine (*Lysistrata* by Aristophanes), who refuses to engage sexually with her warlike husband. And in a more powerful way to many Western audiences, she is exemplified by the first biblical woman, Eve (*The Play of Adam* by Anonymous), who asserts her independence by virtue of disobeying the dominant male authorities. The modern version of this type, however, comes fully into focus with Nora Helmer, the protagonist of Ibsen's *A Doll's House*. Nora is a product of the stifling social conditions in Victorian Europe. Entrapped by gender, husband, and culture, she finally smashes her metaphorical doll house, leaving in ruins the Victorian conception and style of propriety, order, and form. In style Nora heralds the modern realistic protagonist, motivated by inner impulses and needs, and leading to the conception of psychological action developed by Stanislavsky (1936).

Other examples of the liberated wife include Varya (*Summerfolk* by M. Gorki), Lina Szczepanowska (*Misalliance* by G. B. Shaw), Constance Middleton (*The Constant Wife* by W. S. Maugham), and Polly Peachum (*The Threepenny Opera* by B. Brecht and K. Weill).

41.2. Subtype: Castrating Wife

Quality: A third type of wife is adulterous, treacherous, and castrating.

Function: Like the liberated wife, this type will strike out on her own, but in so doing she will first attempt to destroy and often succeed in destroying her husband.

Examples: Clytemnestra (*Agamemnon* by Aeschylus), Queen Isabella (*Edward II* by C. Marlowe), Laura (*The Father* by A. Strindberg), Alice (*The Dance of Death* by A. Strindberg), The Young Woman (*Machinal* by S. Treadwell), and Martha (*Who's Afraid of Virginia Woolf?* by E. Albee).

42. Role Type: Mother-in-Law

Quality: This is generally a comic type—nagging and obnoxious.

Function: She functions as comic relief, shaking up the complacency of the husband–wife relationship, and allowing audiences to laugh at their own burdens from in-laws.

Style: This is generally a stylized character enacted in a broad style.

Examples: Sostrata (*The Mother-in-Law* by Terence), Madame Pernelle (*Tartuffe* by Molière), Signora Frola (*Right You Are (If You Think You Are)* by L. Pirandello), Marfa Ignatyevna Kabanov (*The Storm* by A. Ostrovsky), Maud (*Cloud Nine* by C. Churchill), and Mother (*Barefoot in the Park* by N. Simon).

43. Role Type: Widow/Widower

Quality: This type, which also includes the spinster/bachelor, is marked by being alone and sometimes lonely, other times content and self-contained.

Function: The function of this type is to endure, to make do, to accept the limitations of a life without a spouse.

Examples: Atossa (*The Persians* by Aeschylus), The Old Bachelor (*The Braggart Warrior* by Plautus), Helene Alving (*Ghosts* by H. Ibsen), Olga (*The Three Sisters* by A. Chekhov), Widow Quinn (*The Playboy of the Western World* by J. M. Synge), Mrs. Kendall Frayne (*The Second Man* by S. W. Behrman), Raimunda (*The Passion Flower* by J. Benavente), Charles Condomine (*Blithe Spirit* by N. Coward), Judith (*Judith* by H. Bernstein), and Madame Rosepettle (*Oh Dad, Poor Dad, Mama's Hung You in the Closet and I'm Feeling So Sad* by A. Kopit).

44. Role Type: Father

Quality: The conventional father is masculine, strong, loyal, and protective.

Function: The conventional father protects the family and provides a positive masculine role model.

Style: Although sometimes presented in a stylized fashion, like Abraham in the anonymous medieval morality play *Abraham and Isaac,* the father is generally enacted representationally.

Examples: Hegio (*The Captives* by Plautus), Henry IV (*Henry IV, Parts I and II,* by Shakespeare), Father Day (*Life with Father* by H. Lindsay and R. Crouse), Pa Joad (*The Grapes of Wrath,* adaptation of J. Steinbeck novel by F. Galati).

44.1. Subtype: Tyrannical Father

Quality: This negative version of the father is tyrannical, power-hungry, and morally ambivalent.

Function: His function is to control his family and hold on to power at all costs.

Examples: Agamemnon (*Iphigenia in Aulis* by Euripides), Barabad (*The Jew of Malta* by C. Marlowe), Edward Moulton-Barrett (*The Barretts of Wimpole Street* by R. Besier), Old Mahon (*The Playboy of the Western World* by J. M. Synge), James Tyrone (*Long Day's Journey into Night* by E. O'Neill), and Yekel Shapshowitch (*The God of Vengeance* by S. Asch).

45. Role Type: Husband

Quality: The conventional husband is the breadwinner and provider. He is faithful, protective, loving, and strong.

Function: This type provides for his wife and maintains an aura of strength and stability.

Style: He is generally enacted in a representational style.

Examples: Admetus (*Alcestis* by Euripides), Adam (*The Play of Adam* by Anonymous), John Frankford (*A Woman Killed with Kindness* by T. Heywood), Papa (*I Remember Mama* by J. Van Druten), Nat Miller (*Ah! Wilderness* by E. O'Neill), and Henry (*The Real Thing* by T. Stoppard).

45.1. Subtype: Brutal Husband

Quality: An alternative version of the husband is brutal and unfeeling, often deceptive and adulterous.

Function: This husband satisfies his desires at the expense of his wife.

Examples: Jason (*Medea* by Euripides), Cornwall (*King Lear* by Shakespeare), Sullen (*The Beaux' Strategem* by G. Farquhar), Captain Edgar (*The Dance of Death* by A. Strindberg), and Weston (*Curse of the Starving Class* by S. Shepard).

45.2. Subtype: Weak Husband

Quality: A third version of the husband is weak and insecure, often fearful of women.

Function: This type offers a portrait of the neurotic, ambivalent man, conflicted in his sexuality and relationships to women. His function is to remain fearful, inspiring fear among men of similar propensities in the audience, and to perpetuate a dependence upon the judgment of women.

Examples: Alonzo (*The Changeling* by T. Middleton and W. Rowley), George Tesman (*Hedda Gabler* by H. Ibsen), Captain (*The Father* by A. Strindberg), Myron (*Awake and Sing* by C. Odets), Frank

Elgin (*The Country Girl* by C. Odets), Crocker-Harris (*The Browning Version* by T. Rattigan), George (*Who's Afraid of Virginia Woolf?* by E. Albee), and Ozzie (*Sticks and Bones* by D. Rabe).

46. Role Type: Son

Quality: The conventional son is respectful and loyal, striving to emulate the father.

Function: His goal is to carry on the tradition modeled by the father and to live up to his father's expectations.

Examples: Isaac (*Abraham and Isaac* by Anonymous), Edgar (*King Lear* by Shakespeare), George Gibbs (*Our Town* by T. Wilder), and Eugene Jerome (*Brighton Beach Memoirs* by N. Simon).

46.1. Subtype: Renegade/Rebel Son

Quality: This type is trapped by his family and needs to escape. He is rebellious, sometimes vengeful, hostile, egocentric, and restless.

Function: The renegade son functions to leave home and make his own way in the world, then return home to take over his father's place.

Examples: Haemon (*Antigone* by Sophocles), Henry, Prince of Wales (*Henry IV, Part II* by Shakespeare), Stephen Undershaft (*Major Barbara* by G. B. Shaw), Christy Mahon (*The Playboy of the Western World* by J. M. Synge), The Billionaire's Son (*Gas II* by G. Kaiser), Biff Loman (*Death of a Salesman* by A. Miller), and David (*Sticks and Bones* by D. Rabe).

46.2. Subtype: Bastard Son/Prodigal Son

Quality: This type is a villain to his family. He is manipulative, controlling, sometimes murderous, often illegitimate.

Function: He functions to exploit the family and satisfy his need for power and control.

Examples: Edmund (*King Lear* by Shakespeare), Philip the Bastard (*King John* by Shakespeare), Valentine (*Love for Love* by W. Congreve), Frederico (*Justice Not Revenge* by L. de Vega), Esau (*Jacob's Dream* by R. Beer Hoffmann), and Jamie Tyrone (*Long Day's Journey into Night* by E. O'Neill).

47. Role Type: Daughter

Quality: The conventional daughter is protective of the father. She is generally dutiful, gentle, and nurturing, developing in the image of the mother.

Function: Her function is to stay at home and care for the family; to protect the father and emulate the mother; and to add a sense of grace, beauty, and harmony to the family.

Examples: Ismene (*Antigone* and *Oedipus at Colonus* by Sophocles), Miranda (*The Tempest* by Shakespeare), and Katrin (*Mother Courage and Her Children* by B. Brecht).

47.1. Subtype: Renegade/Rebel Daughter

Quality: This type is rebellious, self-assured, powerful, and independent. She tends to be heroic, often successful in business and sexual matters.

Function: The rebellious daughter breaks from the conventional expectations of the family and satisfies her own professional, ethical, and personal needs.

Examples: Cassandra (*Agamemnon* by Aeschylus), Jessica (*The Merchant of Venice* by Shakespeare), Electra (*Electra* by J. Giraudoux), Rifkele (*The God of Vengeance* by S. Asch), and Alice (*I Never Sang for My Father* by R. Anderson).

47.2. Subtype: Bastard Daughter/Vengeful Daughter

Quality: This type is promiscuous and pariah-like. She lives on the edge of conventionality and needs to prove her legitimacy. At times, she seeks revenge on those blood relatives who she feels have stood in her way.

Function: Her purpose is to prove her worth and legitimacy and to assert her power.

Examples: Regan and Goneril (*King Lear* by Shakespeare), Regine (*Ghosts* by H. Ibsen), Foundling and Marie (*The Daughter of the Regiment* by J. Bayard), Rhoda (*The Bad Seed* by M. Anderson), Claudia Faith Draper (*Nuts* by T. Topor), and Arlene (*Getting Out* by M. Norman).

47.3. Subtype: Daughter in Distress/Daughter as Victim

Quality: A third type of daughter is vulnerable, victimized, cloistered, or held captive against her will.

Function: On the one hand, the victimized daughter submits to the will of the powerful male; on the other, she endures her suffering, on occasion transcending it.

Examples: Iphigenia (*Iphigenia in Aulis* by Euripides), Perdita (*The Winter's Tale* by Shakespeare), Varya (*The Cherry Orchard* by A. Chekhov), Girl (*The Ghost Sonata* by A. Strindberg), Elizabeth Barrett (*The*

Barretts of Wimpole Street by R. Besier), and Chrissy (*In the Boom Boom Room* by D. Rabe).

48. Role Type: Sister

Quality: The conventional sister is supportive of her siblings, compassionate, intelligent, gentle, sometimes deferential to the brother.

Function: The sister supports and unconditionally loves the brother. She serves as a role model for younger sisters and as a companion for older ones.

Style: Although most of the family roles can be played in either presentational and representational ways, this particular type tends to be enacted in a realistic fashion.

Examples: Electra (*Electra* by Euripides), Ismene and Antigone (*Oedipus at Colonus* by Sophocles), Ophelia (*Hamlet* by Shakespeare), Olga, Irina, and Masha (*The Three Sisters* by A. Chekhov), Laura (*The Glass Menagerie* by T. Williams), Ruth (*The Effect of Gamma Rays on Man-in-the-Moon Marigolds* by P. Zindel), and Kate (*Dancing at Lughnasa* by B. Friel).

48.1. Subtype: Renegade/Rebel Sister

Quality: This type of sister is independent and controlling. She tends to be sexual, at times incestuous.

Function: The renegade sister mocks convention. She struggles to get her own needs met within the often stifling bond with her brothers and/or sisters.

Examples: Annabella (*'Tis Pity She's a Whore* by J. Ford), Meg (*Crimes of the Heart* by B. Henley), May (*Fool for Love* by S. Shepard).

49. Role Type: Brother

Quality: The conventional brother is protective of his siblings, strong, loyal, and paternal.

Function: He functions to defend and protect his siblings.

Examples: Orestes (*Electra* by Euripides), Micio and Demea (*The Brothers* by Terence), Abel (*The Play of Adam* by Anonymous), Laertes (*Hamlet* by Shakespeare), Edgar (*King Lear* by Shakespeare), Tom (*The Glass Menagerie* by T. Williams), and Victor (*The Price* by A. Miller).

49.1. Subtype: Renegade/Rebel Brother

Quality: This type of brother is uninterested in acting as a brother to his siblings. He is egocentric and often destructive.

Function: The renegade brother functions to satisfy his own needs, often at the expense of a sibling.

Examples: Polyneices (*The Seven against Thebes* by Aeschylus), Cain (*The Play of Adam* by Anonymous), Oliver (*As You Like It* by Shakespeare), Andrew (*Beyond the Horizon* by E. O'Neill), and Gooper (*Cat on a Hot Tin Roof* by T. Williams).

50. Role Type: Grandparent (see also Elder)

Quality: The grandparent, like the elder, is wise and philosophical, patient and understanding.

Function: This type functions to pass on traditional values to the younger members of the family and to offer a philosophical point of view based on experience and acquired wisdom.

Examples: Peleus (*Andromache* by Euripides), Cadmus (*The Bacchae* by Euripides), Jacob (*Awake and Sing* by C. Odets), Gramps (*On Borrowed Time* by P. Osborn), Grandma (*The American Dream by E. Albee*), Grandmother (*Billy Liar* by K. Waterhouse and W. Hall), Granma and Grampa (*The Grapes of Wrath*, adaptation of J. Steinbeck novel by F. Galati).

50.1. Subtype: Senile or Mad Old Person

Quality: This version of the grandparent is irrational and foolish rather than wise; restricted and confused in thought; either tight and controlled or out of control.

Function: This type confounds and frustrates the young, often providing an offbeat and unconventional sense of whimsy and poetry.

Examples: Strepsiades (*The Clouds* by Aristophanes), King Lear (*King Lear* by Shakespeare), Countess Aurelia (*The Madwoman of Chaillot* by J. Giraudoux), Ephraim Cabot (*Desire under the Elms* by E. O'Neill), Colonel J. C. Kinkaid (*The Last Meeting of the Knights of the White Magnolia* by P. Jones), and Willy Stark (*The Sunshine Boys* by N. Simon).

Classification: POLITICS/GOVERNMENT

51. Role Type: Reactionary

Quality: This political type is backward-looking, extremely conservative and rigid in thought and behavior, often ruthless and brutal in pushing through this point of view.

Function: The reactionary functions to repress those who represent an open, liberal point of view and to subjugate spontaneity and critical thought in the pursuit of that aim.

Examples: Angelo (*Measure for Measure* by Shakespeare), Danforth (*The Crucible* by A. Miller), Michael Marthraun (*Cock-a-Doodle-Dandy* by S. O'Casey), Prince Paul (*Dirty Hands* by J.-P. Sartre), Arthur Goldman (*The Man in the Glass Booth* by R. Shaw), Dictator (*The Best of All Possible Worlds* by A.M. Ballesteros), L. D. Alexander (*The Last Meeting of the Knights of the White Magnolia* by P. Jones), and Aunt Dan (*Aunt Dan and Lemon* by W. Shawn).

52. Role Type: Conservative

Quality: This type is traditional and backward-looking—not as ideologically extreme as the reactionary, yet resisting change and critical of new ideas.

Function: The conservative attempts to preserve the status quo and resist a move into an uncertain future. This type avoids or critiques new ideas and feelings.

Examples: Cinesias (*Lysistrata* by Aristophanes), Montague and Capulet (*Romeo and Juliet* by Shakespeare), Harpagon (*The Miser* by Molière), Torvald (*A Doll's House* by H. Ibsen), Queen Elizabeth (*Mary of Scotland* by M. Anderson), Pobedonsikov (*The Bathhouse* by V. Mayakovsky), Norman Thayer (*On Golden Pond* by E. Thompson), and Mother Miriam Ruth (*Agnes of God* by J. Pielmeir).

52.1. Subtype: Traditionalist

Quality: Another form of conservative maintains faith in the positive values of traditional political, religious, and family life.

Function: This type promulgates and passes on traditional values.

Examples: Hegio (*The Captives* by Plautus), Kate (at the conclusion of *The Taming of the Shrew* by Shakespeare), Grandpa Vanderhof (*You Can't Take It with You* by G. Kaufman and M. Hart), George M. Cohan (*George M.* by M. Stewart, J. Pascal, and F. Pascal), and Tevye (*Fiddler on the Roof* by J. Stein, J. Bock, and S. Harnick).

53. Role Type: Pacifist

Quality: The pacifist is nonviolent and idealistic. This type believes in the perfectibility of humanity and works toward the elimination of armed conflict.

Function: The pacifist wages peace and offers an alternative to war.

Examples: Classical and contemporary examples of the pacifist include Trygaeus and Peace (*Peace* by Aristophanes), Romeo (*Romeo and Juliet* by Shakespeare), Thoreau (*The Night Thoreau Spent in Jail* by J. Lawrence and R. Lee), Lena Younger (*A Raisin in the Sun* by L. Hansberry), and Abbie Hoffman (*The Chicago Conspiracy* by C. Marowitz).

54. Role Type: Revolutionary

Quality: The revolutionary is generally radical, moral, and idealistic, often humorless.

Function: This type rebels against the established order and seeks to replace it with a more humane system as defined by the ideology of the revolutionary.

Examples: Brutus (*Julius Caesar* by Shakespeare), Giovanni (*The Burnt Flower Bed* by U. Betti), The Weavers (*The Weavers* by G. Hauptmann), Pavel (*The Mother* by B. Brecht), Joan Dark (*St. Joan of the Stockyards* by B. Brecht), Dick Dudgeon (*The Devil's Disciple* by G. B. Shaw), Joe Hill (*The Man Who Never Died* by B. Stavis), Malcolm X (*One Day When I Was Lost* by J. Baldwin), and The Maniac and The Journalist (*Accidental Death of an Anarchist* by D. Fo).

54.1. Subtype: Self-Serving Revolutionary

Quality: The revolutionary may also be power-hungry and bloodthirsty, rigid and ruthless, serving a personal need for power rather than a political ideology.

Function: This type usurps power from established leaders for personal gain.

Examples: Cassius (*Julius Caesar* by Shakespeare), Robespierre (*Danton's Death* by G. Buchner), Commissar Amos (*The Queen and the Rebels* by U. Betti), Macbett (*Macbett* by E. Ionesco), Carlos (*Savages* by C. Hampton), and Gethin Price (*Comedians* by T. Griffiths).

55. Role Type: Head of State

Quality: This type, exemplified by a king or queen, is regal, aristocratic, powerful, privileged, and either benevolent or despotic (or some combination of both).

Function: The head of state rules those of a lower status and serves as a symbol of power and order.

Examples: Oedipus (*Oedipus Rex* by Sophocles), Julius Caesar (*Julius Caesar* by Shakespeare), King of Rhodes (*The Maid's Tragedy* by F. Beaumont and J. Fletcher), King Philip II (*The Mayor of Zalamea* by P. Calderon), Elizabeth (*Elizabeth the Queen* by M. Anderson), Mary, Queen of Scots (*Maria Stuart* by F. Schiller, *Mary and the Executioner* by W. Hildesheimer), Winston Churchill (*Soldiers* by R. Hochhuth).

56. Role Type: Minister/Advisor/Councillor

Quality: This type is subservient and deferential, yet politically wise and often shrewd, smug, and controlling.

Function: The councillor runs a certain department within the state, offering advice when requested and deferring to those in positions of authority. Yet this astute type also controls considerable power, and knows how to manipulate the head of state and the system in order to assert that power.

Examples: Tranio (*The Haunted House* by Plautus), Polonius (*Hamlet* by Shakespeare), Armostes (*The Broken Heart* by J. Ford), The Minister of Repression (*The Best of All Possible Worlds* by A. M Ballesteros).

56.1. Subtype: Moral Minister

Quality: Some ministers are moral and principled, offering opinions on political matters even when their opinions are unpopular with those in greater power.

Function: This kind of minister offers advice based upon a critical assessment of the political situation and a personal moral philosophy; he often risks his personal safety in advancing an opinion contradictory to that of a head of state.

Style: This alternative version of the minister is generally presented in a realistic fashion.

Examples: Tiresias (*Oedipus Rex* by Sophocles), Escalus (*Measure for Measure* by Shakespeare), Burrhus (*Britannicus* by J. Racine), Thomas More (*A Man for All Seasons* by R. Bolt), Thomas Becket (*Becket* by J. Anouilh).

57. Role Type: Bureaucrat

Quality: The bureaucrat as a role type is efficient, dull, fastidious, conventional, bourgeois, and small in status.

Function: This type is a clerk who functions to keep the books, maintain a sense of order, and focus upon the minutiae of life, often missing the forest for the trees.

Style: This is generally a presentational character—a cipher or symbol of one lost in a bureacracy yet responsible for maintaining it.

Examples: Dapper (*The Alchemist* by B. Jonson), Cashier (*From Morn to Midnight* by G. Kaiser), Chief Clerk (*The Trial*, adaptation of F. Kafka novel by J. L. Barrault), Zoditch (*Journey of the Fifth Horse* by R. Ribman).

Classification: LEGAL

58. Role Type: Lawyer

Quality: The lawyer is protective, moral, and intelligent.

Function: The lawyer's job is to defend and protect those who have been falsely accused.

Style: Lawyers are generally enacted realistically.

Example: Bdelycleon (*The Wasps* by Aristophanes), Portia (*The Merchant of Venice* by Shakespeare), Mr. Poskit and Mr. Bellamy (*The Magistrate* by A. W. Pinero), Henry Drummond (*Inherit the Wind* by J. Lawrence and R. Lee), Otis Baker and Louis Schade (*The Andersonville Trial* by S. Levitt), Quentin (*After the Fall* by A. Miller), William Kunstler (*The Chicago Conspiracy* by C. Marowitz), and Aaron Levinsky (*Nuts* by T. Topor).

58.1. Subtype: Greedy Lawyer

Quality: An alternative view of the lawyer is one who is greedy, amoral, and self-serving.

Function: This version of the lawyer manipulates justice for his own ends.

Examples: Pierre Patelin (*Pierre Patelin* by Anonymous), Voltore (*Volpone* by B. Jonson), Cribbs (*The Drunkard* by W. Smith), Mr. Sharp (*Money* by E. Bulwer-Lytton), Bill Maitland (*Inadmissible Evidence* by J. Osborne), and Roy Cohn (*Angels in America* by T. Kushner).

59. Role Type: Judge

Quality: The moral judge is impartial and fair, authoritative and dispassionate, wise and judicious.

Function: This judge functions to render impartial judgments based upon empirical evidence, to punish criminal acts, and to maintain order.

Examples: Athena (*The Eumenides* by Aeschylus), Daemones (*The Rope* by Plautus), Duke of Venice (*The Merchant of Venice* by Shakespeare), Vergil (*The Poetaster* by B. Jonson), Azdak (*The Caucasian Chalk Circle* by B. Brecht), Judge Cust and the Chief Justice (*Cor-*

ruption in the Palace of Justice by U. Betti), Presiding Judge (*The Man in the Glass Booth* by R. Shaw), Lieutenant Commander Challee (*The Caine Mutiny Court-Martial* by H. Wouk), and Chairman (*Are You Now or Have You Ever Been?* by E. Bentley).

59.1. Subtype: Immoral Judge

Quality: An alternative version of the judge is one who is immoral and unjudicious, punitive and biased, self-serving or in the service of a repressive state.

Function: This immoral judge functions to punish unfairly, serving personal and/or political aims rather than justice.

Examples: Robert Shallow (*The Merry Wives of Windsor* by Shakespeare), Judge Von Weghahn (*The Beaver Coat* by G. Hauptmann), Danforth (*The Crucible* by A. Miller), and Judge Hoffman (*The Chicago Conspiracy* by C. Marowitz).

60. Role Type: Defendant

Quality: This type is defensive, self-protective, and often self-righteous. The defendant is sometimes guilty, but most times is anxious to be proven innocent and to be exonerated.

Function: Defendants function to protest their indictments and to prove their innocence.

Style: Generally defendants are portrayed representationally.

Examples: Orestes (*The Eumenides* by Aeschylus), Antonio (*The Merchant of Venice* by Shakespeare), Coolie (*The Exception and the Rule* by B. Brecht), Joan of Arc (*Saint Joan* by G. B. Shaw), Cates (*Inherit the Wind* by J. Lawrence and R. Lee), Henry Wirz (*The Andersonville Trial* by S. Levitt), J. Robert Oppenheimer (*In the Matter of J. Robert Oppenheimer* by H. Kipphardt), Ethel and Julius Rosenberg (*Inquest* by D. Freed), The Chicago Seven (*The Chicago Conspiracy* by C. Marowitz).

61. Role Type: Jury (see also Chorus)

Quality: The jury is a representative sample of a community, usually impartial and fair, sometimes in the service of the state.

Function: The jury functions to offer an impartial collective judgment based upon empirical evidence.

Examples: Philocleon and the Wasps (*The Wasps* by Aristophanes), Twelve Athenians (*The Eumenides* by Aeschylus), The Inquisition (*Galileo* by B. Brecht), The Control Chorus (*The Measures Taken* by B. Brecht), Jury (*Inherit the Wind* by J. Lawrence and R. Lee).

62. Role Type: Witness

Quality: This type is an onlooker, often definitive and righteous, who expresses a particular point of view. The witness is biased in favor of either the guilt or innocence of a defendant.

Function: Witnesses offer a specific point of view to a judge or jury, based upon first-hand knowledge; they have viewed an event from a safe distance without getting directly involved.

Style: Like other role types involved in judicial matters, the witness is generally a realistically drawn character.

Examples: A Herdsman (*Oedipus Rex* by Sophocles), Crispinus (*The Poetaster* by B. Jonson), The Four Agitators (*The Measures Taken* by B. Brecht), Rachel (*Inherit the Wind* by J. Lawrence and R. Lee), Lieutenant Colonel Chandler (*The Andersonville Trial* by S. Levitt), David Greenglass (*Inquest* by D. Freed), and Allen Ginsberg (*The Chicago Conspiracy Trial* by R. Sossi).

63. Role Type: Prosecutor/Inquisitor

Quality: This type is aggressive, self-righteous, ruthless, and driven, committed to proving the guilt of the defendant.

Function: The prosecutor's aim is to prosecute, sometimes unrelentingly, in order to prove to judge and jury the unequivocal guilt of a defendant. The inquisitor often forces the defendant into a confession of guilt.

Examples: Pontius Pilate (*The Passion Play* by Anonymous), the Inquisitor (*Saint Joan* by G. B. Shaw), Inquisitor (*Galileo* by B. Brecht), Matthew Brady (*Inherit the Wind* by J. Lawrence and R. Lee), Lieutenant Colonel N. P. Chipman (*The Andersonville Trial* by S. Levitt), Cromwell (*A Man for All Seasons* by R. Bolt), and Franklin Macmillan (*Nuts* by T. Topor).

Classification: Socioeconomic Status

64. Role Type: Lower Class (see also Pariah)

Quality: A long way from the intellectual privilege of the critic and the social privilege of the aristocrat lies the lower-class role type. This is the domain of the beggar and peasant, the downtrodden, squalid, and oppressed. This type, poor in material possessions and sometimes in spirit, is oppressed, neglected, and invisible to those with plenty. Sometimes depressed, the lower class type may also be ironic and witty, rising above the physical squalor.

Function: The function of the lower-class role type is, on the one hand, to express the conditions and consequences of poverty; and, on the other, to endure, sometimes with a touch of irony and mockery at those whom Shaw might call "the undeserving rich." Furthermore, this type draws attention to the connection between material and spiritual poverty, and challenges the human spirit to transcend the conditions of economic oppression.

Examples: In the 18th century, J. Gay dramatized the life of this class in *The Beggar's Opera*, later to be revised by B. Brecht and K. Weill for greater political effect as *The Threepenny Opera*. Modern portraits of this class are found in M. Gorki's sordid inhabitants of *The Lower Depths* and in G. B. Shaw's Alfred P. Doolittle in *Pygmalion*, a prime example of "the undeserving poor." This latter example adds the qualities of irony and wit to one who would otherwise live a squalid existence. Other examples throughout the ages include Charlotte and Francisco (*Don Juan or the Statue at the Feast* by Molière), Men and Women of the People (*Danton's Death* by G. Büchner), Coolies (*The Measures Taken* by B. Brecht), Beggars (*The Golem* by H. Leivik), and The Matchseller (*A Slight Ache* by H. Pinter).

65. Role Type: Working Class/Worker

Quality: This type is unpretentious and plain-speaking, earthy, uneducated and unsophisticated, diligent, underpaid and unrewarded. Many working-class characters also appear as uncultured, ignorant, and servile. The worker tends to be traditional and conservative in values.

Function: The function of this group is to work hard at a minimal wage for the good of the family or state. An early conception of the worker role was that of the ignoramus who existed for the pleasure and ridicule of his patrons.

Style: Hardly a threat to the ruling class, the early workers found in Renaissance plays amused their audiences in a stylized form of low comedy later to become popularized in music halls and burlesque theatres throughout much of the world. In modern productions, the worker type appears in a more representational form.

Examples: During the Renaissance, the voices of the working class started to be heard in the theatre. In *A Midsummer Night's Dream,* Shakespeare introduces the mechanicals, lowly workers moonlighting as amateur actors, who are hired to amuse the court. The troupe of Bottom the weaver, Snug the joiner, Quince the carpenter, and the others represents a view of the world as organized by class and status. The masses are very much portrayed as asses in this play. Other examples include Three Shepherds (*The Second Shepherd's Play* by Anonymous), Mistress Quickly (*Henry IV, Part 1* by Shakespeare), Eliza Doolittle (*Pygmalion* by G. B. Shaw), Beatie Bryant (*Roots* by A. Wesker), Val and Shirley (*Fen* by C. Churchill), and Troy (*Fences* by A. Wilson).

65.1. Subtype: Brutal Worker

Quality: The worker may also be portrayed as frustrated, brutal, and insensitive.

Function: This alternative worker acts out frustrations violently, often proving injurious to an intimate or to himself.

Examples: The worker role expanded considerably as the Western world moved directly into the Industrial Revolution. The bumbling mechanical gave way to the frustrated worker burdened with too many pressures and too little money, who acts out brutally against family and society. In contemporary drama, this type is well represented in the squalid, cruel working-class figures created by the German playwright F. X. Kroetz, such as Otto in *Through the Leaves*. Other examples include Juvan (*The Goat Song* by F. Werfel), Mattern the Mason (*Hannele* by G. Hauptmann), Barabbas (*Barabbas* by M. de Ghelderode), Brutus Jones (*The Emperor Jones* by E. O'Neill), Lin To (*The Good Woman of Setzuan* by B. Brecht), and Boze (*The Petrified Forest* by R. Sherwood).

65.2. Subtype: Revolutionary Worker

Quality: Earthy and underpaid, yet radical, this type represents the worker as revolutionary.

Function: The revolutionary worker's function is to rebel against the established order, joining with fellow workers in radical activity.

Examples: In the late 19th century, an image appeared of the protelarian as revolutionary, inspired by the writings of Karl Marx and well represented in the early plays of Brecht. Modern examples of this type include Billionaire–Worker (*Gas II* by G. Kaiser), Young Comrade (*The Measures Taken* by B. Brecht), Agate (*Waiting for Lefty* by C. Odets), and Tom Joad (*The Grapes of Wrath*, adaptation of J. Steinbeck novel by F. Galati).

66. Role Type: Middle Class

Quality: This type is conventional in morality and sensibility, respectable, colorless, and generally apolitical.

Function: The middle-class role type functions to uphold the conventions of the dominant culture, to do and think the expected, and to defend against the encroachment of intellectual and ethical challenge. Furthermore, this type serves a satirical function, poking fun at the materialistic values and petty aspirations of the bourgeoisie.

Examples: Charisius (*The Arbitration* by Menander), Arnolphe (*The School for Wives* by Molière), M. Perrichon (*The Voyage of M. Perrichon* by E. Labiche), Consul Bernick (*Pillars of Society* by H. Ibsen), Moll (*The Burgomaster* by G. Hofmann), Christian Maske (*The Snob* by K. Sternheim), Mr. and Mrs. Smith (*The Bald Soprano* by E. Ionesco), and Peter (*The Zoo Story* by E. Albee).

66.1. Subtype: Nouveau Riche

Quality: With the rise of the bourgeoisie in 17th-century France, Molière presented his own satirical version of a fairly new role type, well exemplified by M. Jourdain, the title character of *The Would-Be Gentleman*. This nouveau riche is upwardly mobile, pretentious, and foolish in the attempt to acquire culture and status.

Function: The nouveau riche plays the simpleton and offers a satirical view of the consequences of reaching beyond one's grasp.

Style: Such a satirical function often suggests a presentational style of performance, allowing the audience members enough distance to laugh at their own tendencies toward pretentiousness.

Examples: The classical M. Jourdain gives way to such other characters as Mr. and Mrs. Tiffany (*Fashion* by A. C. Mowatt), Egor Bulychov (*Egor Bulychov and the Others* by M. Gorki), Ronald and Marion (*Absurd Person Singular* by A. Ayckbourn), Michael, Phillip, and Lisa (*Key Exchange* by K. Wade), and Stephen (*Eastern Standard* by R. Greenberg).

66.2. Subtype: Merchant/Salesperson

Quality: The merchant is average, gregarious, and extroverted, a hustler and glad-hander. This type stakes self-worth on the quantity of sales.

Function: The function of the merchant is to sell a product through selling his/her personality.

Style: Although often an emblem—as A. Miller's Willy Loman (*Death of a Salesman*) is the symbolic "low man" —this type is generally enacted in an emotional, realistic fashion.

Examples: Other examples include Antonio (*The Merchant of Venice* by Shakespeare), Venturewell (*The Knight of the Burning Pestle* by F. Beaumont and J. Fletcher), Lopahin (*The Cherry Orchard* by A. Chekhov), and Hickey (*The Iceman Cometh* by E. O'Neill).

66.3. Subtype: Usurer

Quality: An alternative type of merchant is a usurer: ruthless, miserly, and exploitative.

Function: This type exploits customers and plays more the deceiver and miser than the gregarious businessperson.

Style: This type tends to be portrayed in a presentational style.

Examples: Shylock (*The Merchant of Venice* by Shakespeare), Merchant (*The Exception and the Rule* by B. Brecht), Marco Polo (*Marco Millions* by E. O'Neill), and Uncle Fatso (*The Difficult Life of Uncle Fatso* by P. Schumann).

67. Role Type: Upper Class

Quality: The upper-class role type is that of privilege, wealth, power, and superiority.

Function: In function, the upper-class role exists to assert the power that comes from wealth and opportunity.

Style: The upper-class role type extends throughout drama in various forms that include satire (e.g., in the hands of the Restoration playwrights) and psychological realism (e.g., in the more modern musings of Chekhov, as he surveyed the decline of the Russian nobility).

Examples: As Molière often focused his barbs on the middle class, the British Restoration playwrights aimed at the pretensions of the upper crust. We find in the plays of Congreve, Etherege, and Farquhar, among others, a witty depiction of the privileged and leisured classes, who seem to spend all their time scheming and talking. Examples include Dorimant (*The Man of Mode* by G. Etherege), Madame Ranevskaya (*The Cherry Orchard* by A. Chekhov), Lord Loam (*The Admirable Crichton* by J. M. Barrie), Victor and Sybil (*Private Lives* by N. Coward), and Father (*The Dining Room* by A. J. Gurney).

67.1. Subtype: Industrialist/Entrepreneur

Quality: This modern subtype of the upper class is the self-made, hard-driving, hard-fisted captain of industry who bears a striking resemblance to the 19th-century American robber barons (exemplified by Cornelius Vanderbilt) and later venture capitalists motivated by a lust for power and wealth. This type is sometimes self-satsified, but more often despondent and controlling.

Function: This type functions to maintain the trappings of power and authority in the workplace and at home.

Examples: Ibsen presented two powerful examples of the industrialist in Solness, the title character of *The Master Builder,* and John Gabriel Borkman, the megalomaniacal financier in the play bearing his name. Other examples of this type include Sir Giles Overreach (*A New Way to Pay Old Debts* by P. Massinger), The Billionaire (*The Coral* by G. Kaiser), Andrew Undershaft (*Major Barbara* by G. B. Shaw), Herr Puntilla (*Herr Puntilla and His Chauffeur Matti* by B. Brecht), Leonie Frothingham (*End of Summer* by S. N. Behrman), Mister Mister (*The Cradle Will Rock* by M. Blitzstein), and Lawrence Garfield (*Other People's Money* by J. Sterner).

67.2. Subtype: Socialite

Quality: This type is wealthy and idle, extravagant and elegant, witty, vapid, and frivolous.

Function: This type indulges in abundant material and cultural pleasures.

Style: Generally the socialite is portrayed in a presentational style.

Examples: Sir Fopling Flutter (*The Man of Mode* by G. Etherege), Algernon Moncrieff (*The Importance of Being Earnest* by O. Wilde), Lady Kitty (*The Circle* by W. S. Maugham), Truman Capote (*Tru* by J. Presson Allen), and Nora Charles (*Nick and Nora* by A. Laurents).

67.3. Subtype: Servant to the Rich

Quality: This type is a form of aristocratic fool—servile and snobbish, sometimes witty, privileged among servants, and highly protective of superiors.

Function: Servants protect the self-importance of the upper classes.

Style: This type is primarily played with high style.

Examples: Xanthias (*The Frogs* by Aristophanes), Oswald (*King Lear* by Shakespeare), Waitwell (*The Way of the World* by W. Congreve), Merriman (*The Importance of Being Earnest* by O. Wilde), Prince Alexandrovitch and Grand Duchess Petrovna (*Tovarich* by J. Deval), and Norman (*The Dresser* by R. Harwood).

68. Role Type: Pariah (see also Lost One and Lower Class)

Quality: Pariahs may be those of noble birth who have violated the political, social, or moral order. Or they may be thrust into their role by virtue of their physical, socioeconomic, political, or moral status. The pariah in theatre may be king or criminal, revolutionary or beggar. The qualities common to all are rejection by their peers and assignment to the fringes of society.

Function: The pariah functions as a challenge to the established order—a warning and reminder that all is not well, and that each gain in life is the other side of a loss. The pariah is often the scapegoat who painfully reminds thoughtful onlookers that they too could easily experience a reversal of fortune.

Examples: The pariah role includes the presentationally drawn classical figures of Oedipus and Lear, and the more contemporary, poetically naturalistic petty thieves, drifters, and cowboys sketched by D. Mamet and S. Shepard. Specific examples include Philoctetes (*Philoctetes* by Sophocles), Shylock (*The Merchant of Venice* by Shakespeare), Peachum (*The Beggar's Opera* by J. Gay), Anna, the Baron, Nastya, et al. (*The Lower Depths* by M. Gorki), Harry Heegan (*The Silver Tassie* by S. O'Casey), Judge, General, and Bishop (*The Balcony* by J. Genet), Hoss (*The Tooth of Crime* by S. Shepard), Rita Joe (*The Ecstasy of Rita Joe* by G. Ryga), Clark Davis (*Short Eyes* by M. Piñero), and Jimmy Rosehips (*A Prayer for My Daughter* by T. Babe).

69. Role Type: Chorus, the Voice of the People

Quality: The creation of the chorus was a major innovation in Greek drama. This role type represents the voice of the people, a collective role later to take a clear moral tone in the medieval character of Everyman. The chorus is lyrical and poetic, though sometimes spoken in a more prosaic vernacular. It is witty, expressive of conventional wisdom and morality, and on occasion critical of the established order.

Function: Several functions of the chorus include (1) generally, to assert a collective voice, the point of view of the common person, or that of the audience; (2) to serve as a foil or challenge to the protagonist; (3) to comment upon the action in an ironic or critical fashion; and (4) to entertain through providing a lyrical interlude, which often heightens the emotional quality of the drama.

Style: The chorus in performance is a highly stylized and thus presentational convention in both classical and modern drama. It is an indispensable part of opera and musical theatre, and such expressionistic playwrights as Brecht have employed various choruses, narrators, and streetsingers to great effect.

Examples: Among the many classical Greek choruses are those of frogs, birds, clouds, and wasps in the plays of the same names by

Aristophanes. Other examples of the chorus include Everyman (*Everyman* by Anonymous), The Chorus (*Henry V* by Shakespeare), Chorus of Canterbury Women (*Murder in the Cathedral* by T. S. Eliot), The Common Man (*A Man for All Seasons* by R. Bolt), and the many choruses within musical theatre (from early opera to such commercial spectacles as *The Phantom of the Opera* and *Miss Saigon*).

Classification: AUTHORITY AND POWER

70. Role Type: Warrior

Quality: This generic type of victor is aggressive, assertive, and moral. Warriors know what they want and are willing to fight to get it, both on the battlefield and on the home front.

Function: The warrior functions to engage in physical, moral, or intellectual battle to defeat an opponent and achieve a specified goal.

Examples: Dicaeopolis (*The Acharnians* by Aristophanes), Rosalind (*As You Like It* by Shakespeare), Goetz von Berlichingen (*Goetz von Berlichingen* by J. W. von Goethe), Adolf (*The Captain* by A. Strindberg), Pizarro and Atahualpa (*The Royal Hunt of the Sun* by P. Shaffer), and Archbishop Oscar Romero (*The Resurrection of Archbishop Oscar Romero of El Salvador* by P. Schumann).

70.1. Subtype: Soldier

Quality: The soldier, also featured in many plays as the captain, is disciplined and warlike. This type is controlled and gallant in peacetime, but violent and murderous in war.

Function: The function of the soldier is to defeat the enemy and defend the state.

Examples: Odysseus (*The Cyclops* by Euripides), Henry V (*Henry V* by Shakespeare), Cyrano de Bergerac (*Cyrano de Bergerac* by E. Rostand), Kragler (*Drums in the Night* by B. Brecht), Billy Bishop (*Billy Bishop Goes to War* by J. Gray), Captain Isaac Whitaker (*A Few Good Men* by A. Sorkin).

70.2. Subtype: Cowardly Soldier (see also Braggart Warrior)

Quality: Acutally a subtype of the soldier, this character is insecure and fearful, sometimes displaying a false sense of bravado.

Function: The cowardly soldier defends against a fear of weakness and failure by joining the military and attempting to impress others.

Style: This type is generally presentational in performance.

Examples: (see also examples under 33.1, Chapter Nine): Pavlo Hummel (*The Basic Training of Pavlo Hummel* by D. Rabe), Billy and Ritchie (*Streamers* by D. Rabe).

70.3. Subtype: Tyrant

Quality: This type of warrior is purposefully assertive, despotic, and power-hungry. The tryant tends to be immoral and megalomaniacal, physically and/or psychologically harmful to others or to self.

Function: The tyrant strives not only to control others, but to brutalize and humiliate them in order to feel powerful.

Style: This type is usually played in a stylized fashion.

Examples: In Renaissance drama, high-born soldiers and statesmen often overstep their authority in their quest for power. Thus we find many examples of the aggressive tyrant, such as Shakespeare's Richard III and Marlowe's Tamburlaine in the plays of the same names. Further examples include Menedemus (*The Self-Tormentor* by Terence), Nero (*Britannicus* by J. Racine), Fernando Gomez de Guzman (*The Sheep Well* by Lope de Vega), Caligula (*Caligula* by A. Camus), Crown (*Porgy* by D. Heyward), John Claggart (*Billy Budd,* adaptation of H. Melville story by L. Coxe and R. Chapman), Head Nurse Ratched (*One Flew over the Cuckoo's Nest,* adaptation of K. Kesey novel by D. Wasserman), Juan Peron (*Evita* by T. Rice and A. Lloyd Webber), and Sister Mary Ignatius (*Sister Mary Ignatius Explains It All for You* by C. Durang).

71. Role Type: Police

Quality: This role type is authoritarian and officious; tough and aggressive; sometimes corrupt, sometimes moral.

Function: The police officer functions to maintain law and order within a community and to arrest and foil real and potential criminals, sometimes using his/her authority for profit.

Examples: The Guard (*Antigone* by Sophocles), Elbow (*Measure for Measure* by Shakespeare), Lockit (*The Beggar's Opera* by J. Gay), Blick and Krupp (*The Time of Your Life* by W. Saroyan), Police Chief (*The Balcony* by J. Genet), Salzer (*The Deputy* by R. Hochhuth), Officer Krupke (*West Side Story* by A. Laurents, S. Sondheim, and L. Bernstein), Police (*Accidental Death of an Anarchist* by D. Fo), Jack and Kelly (*A Prayer for My Daughter* by T. Babe), and Lieutenant Fine (*Clare* by A. Miller).

71.1. Subtype: Clownish Cop

Quality: A popular alternative in dramatic literature is the cop who is foolish, incompetent, and bumbling in the effort to fight crime.

Function: This bumbler functions to poke fun at the power and authority of the police.

Style: The bumbling, clowish cop appears in a presentational style.

Examples: Dogberry (*Much Ado about Nothing* by Shakespeare), The Police (*The Pirates of Penzance* by W. S. Gilbert and A. Sullivan), Police (*Arsenic and Old Lace* by J. Kesselring), and Creep (*Pantagleize* by M. de Ghelderode).

72. Role Type: Killer

Quality: The killer or assassin is violent, passive and/or aggressive, and immoral, resorting to committing murder as a method of resolving conflicts.

Function: This type functions to resolve a personal or political dilemma through a violent act of murder.

Examples: Clytemnestra and Aegisthus (*Agamemnon* by Aeschylus), Macbeth and Lady Macbeth (*Macbeth* by Shakespeare), Aaron the Moor (*Titus Andronicus* by Shakespeare), the Cardinal and the Duke of Calabria (*The Duchess of Malfi* by J. Webster), Yerma (*Yerma* by F. Garcia Lorca), Sweeney Todd (*Sweeney Todd* by G. Pitt), Cain (*Back to Methusaleh* by G. B. Shaw), Hugo (*Dirty Hands* by J.-P. Sartre), The Stranger (*Balm in Gilead* by L. Wilson), and Lee Harvey Oswald (*Assassins* by J. Lapine and S. Sondheim).

72.1. Subtype: Suicide

Quality: The self-killer is passive, fearful, trapped, despondent, and hopeless.

Function: The suicide commits self-murder as a means of escaping from life or punishing the living.

Examples: Ajax (*Ajax* by Sophocles), Ophelia (*Hamlet* by Shakespeare), Hedwig (*The Wild Duck* by H. Ibsen), Julie (*Miss Julie* by A. Strindberg), Treplev (*The Sea Gull* by A. Chekhov), Cho-Cho-San (*Madame Butterfly* by D. Belasco), and Jessie Cates (*'Night, Mother* by M. Norman).

72.2. Subtype: Matricide, Parricide, Infanticide, Fratricide

Quality: This type of killer is amoral, irrational, violent, and in violation of a sacred taboo—the murder of a blood relative (mother, father, child, brother, or sister).

Function: This type seeks to avenge through murder a perceived wrong perpetrated by a blood relative.

Examples: Orestes and Electra (*The Libation Bearers* by Aeschylus), Atreus (*Thyestes* by Seneca), Claudius (*Hamlet* by Shakespeare), Athaliah (*Athaliah* by J. Racine), Cuchulain (*The Only Jealousy of Emer* by W. B. Yeats), and Abbie Putnam (*Desire under the Elms* by E. O'Neill).

In some cases, these murderers are unaware that they have killed a blood relative. When brought to awareness, they must face the profound psychological and moral consequences of the deed. Examples of such murderers include Oedipus (*Oedipus Rex* by Sophocles), Agave (*The Bacchae* by Euripides), Martha (*Cross Purpose* by A. Camus), and Agnes (*Agnes of God* by J. Pielmeir).

CHAPTER ELEVEN

The Taxonomy:
Spiritual and Aesthetic Domains

DOMAIN: SPIRITUAL

Classification: NATURAL BEINGS

73. Role Type: Hero

Quality: The hero journeys forth on a spiritual search that proves in some way to be transformational. This type is moral, inquisitive, and open to confronting the unknown. The classical tragic heroes are those who search for a meaning just beyond their grasp, willing to confront the hardships of the journey and to accept the tragic consequences that arise from uncovering certain elemental ambivalences of being.

Function: Thus, the function of the hero is to take a risky spiritual and psychological journey toward understanding and transformation.

Style: The tragic hero tends to appear in classical drama in a presentational style: in Greek drama, elevated through stilts, masks, and poetic diction; in Renaissance drama, married to the given poetic and stylized conventions of speech and gesture. The modern hero, however, tends to be portrayed more within the tradition of psychological realism. As such, this hero's language and gesture tend to be more naturalistic and less symbolic.

Examples: Antigone (versions of *Antigone* by Sophocles, B. Brecht, and J. Anouilh), Othello (*Othello* by Shakespeare), Mary Stuart (*Maria Stuart* by F. Schiller), Phaedra (*Phaedra* by J. Racine), Abe Lincoln (*Abe Lincoln in Illinois* by R. Sherwood), Quentin (*After the Fall* by A. Miller), Jack Jefferson (*The Great White Hope* by H. Sackler), Fefu (*Fefu and Her Friends* by M. I. Fornes).

73.1. Subtype: Superman

Quality: This type, referring to the notion of a human being striving toward perfection, is infinitely inquisitive, restless, energetic, assertive, and creative. This role type becomes the embodiment of the romantic notion of the search for the exotic and the beautiful, as well as for ultimate knowledge and power.

Function: The function of the superman is to assert the romantic quest to the extreme. This persona, however, is not that of the dreamer or the escapist, but of one who actively pursues greater knowledge and power, who pushes beyond all psychological and moral limits.

Style: This type appears in the presentational style.

Examples: The clearest example is the Faust character as drawn by Marlowe (*Doctor Faustus*) and Goethe (*Faust*), who is consumed by his megalomaniacal search for wisdom. Ibsen depicts the quest for power of his superman-like searchers, Peer Gynt and John Gabriel Borkman. In a play within his *Man and Superman,* G. B. Shaw presents his ironic version of the superman—a Don Juan in hell who will ultimately choose heaven as his final paradise. Following Goethe's version of Faust, other modern examples include Faustus (*Mon Faust* by P. Valéry) and Young, Middle Age, and Old Faust (*Dr. Faustus Lights the Lights* by G. Stein).

73.2. Subtype: Antihero (see also Lost One)

Quality: Whereas the hero journeys forth on a spiritual search, the antihero stays put or moves within very limited psychological territory. Antiheroes are marked by inertia, boredom, and minimal goals. This modern figure is the antithesis of the tragic hero—an ordinary person trapped in ordinary, often dull circumstances.

Function: Antiheroes are small, low men and women, lost in an overwhelmingly indifferent universe. Yet somehow, the antihero endures. Even with the suicide of Willy Loman (*Death of a Salesman* by A. Miller), one feels that a recognition has occurred within his family. His life has had some purpose, at least in the eyes of his wife and son, Biff.

Examples: Other examples include Vanya (*Uncle Vanya* by A. Chekhov), Ham and Clov (*Endgame* by S. Beckett), Berenger (*Rhinoceros* by E. Ionesco), Stephen (*When You Coming Home, Red Ryder* by M. Medoff).

73.3. Subtype: Postmodern Antihero

Quality: The notion of human being as machine was ushered in during the early part of the 20th century by the Russian constructivists and Italian modernists, among others. The postmodern theatre moves further afield, depicting the person as sign, whose meaning can be extracted in as many ways as there are minds to read it. The postmodern role is deconstructed, turned inside out, transformed into a kind of theatrical technology. This extreme form of antihero is an emblem, a cipher, a factotum, with few recognizable human qualities.

Function: The postmodern role functions as an abstract or surrealistic painting; it delights primarily in its form. It is thus, for the most part, devoid of content and of the dramatic unities of time, place, and action. Presenting its themes obtusely, it alienates its viewers not only from their feelings, but also from their thoughts. This is theatre on the other side of Brecht—a theatre of perception rather than criticism.

Style: The furthest abstraction of role in the 20th century is that which appears in postmodern forms of theatre and performance art. The role becomes one of many formal elements in the production, often assuming equal status with sets, lights, and sound. For the most part, all notion of character development is absent. This is a theatre of form, not of content.

Examples: The large theatrical canvases painted by R. Wilson, for example, appear to be more in the tradition of the visual than of the performance arts. The stage images are pictures that move in small increments of time and space: an actor creeping across the front of the stage over a period of 5 minutes, a group of actors slowly moving their heads from side to side in synchrony. Characters are named in Wilson's theatre pieces—Einstein, Stalin, Lincoln, Freud—but they serve more as icons than as roles, visual cues to a deconstructed puzzle of images that exist together without quite fitting.

P. Schumann, in The Bread and Puppet Theatre, prefers to hide the actor altogether behind a mask or within a giant puppet. In his sculptural, political, and spiritual theatre, there is little use for the human actor. His figures are types with names like the Diagonal Man and the Washerwomen.

Other examples include Rhoda (*Rhoda in Potatoland* by R. Foreman), Rosencrantz and Guildenstern (*Rosencrantz and Guildenstern Are Dead* by T. Stoppard), Hamlet and Ophelia (*Hamletmachine* by H. Müller), and Swedenborg (*Swedenborg* by Ping Chong).

74. Role Type: Visionary (see also Wise Person and Appollonian God/Goddess)

Quality: This type, inclusive of the prophet and seer, is characterized by prophetic wisdom, insight, and clairvoyance.

Function: The visionary sees beyond external events and draws conclusions based upon insight and clairvoyance. This type predicts the future on the basis of such spiritual knowing.

Style: The visionary is generally enacted in a presentational style.

Examples: Tiresias, the blind prophet in *Oedipus Rex* by Sophocles, is the only one in Thebes capable of envisioning the truth of the identity and fate of Oedipus. Cassandra is portrayed by Euripides in *The Trojan Women* as also capable of predicting the tragic fate that awaits Agamemnon on his return home from the Trojan War.

Other examples include Soothsayer (*Julius Caesar* by Shakespeare), Princess Kail (*War, a Te Deum* by C. Hauptmann), Sir Henry Harcourt-Reilly (*The Cocktail Party* by T. S. Eliot), Joan (*The Lark* by J. Anouilh), Madame Arcati (*Blithe Spirit* by N. Coward), Charles Lacy (*The Water Engine* by D. Mamet), and Mother Ann Lee and Mary Wollstonecraft (*Making Peace: A Fantasy* by K. Malpede).

75. Role Type: Orthodox

Quality: The orthodox is a highly moral believer, fully committed to a single belief system, which serves as a dogma.

Function: The orthodox believes fully in the principles of a single faith, practicing its rituals and receiving sustenance from its teachings.

Examples: Abraham (*Abraham and Isaac* by Anonymous), Job (*The Book of Job* by Anonymous), J. B. (*J. B.* by A. MacLeish), Thomas Becket (*Murder in the Cathedral* by T. S. Eliot), Rubashov (*Darkness at Noon* by S. Kingsley), Father Duquesne (*The First Legion* by E. Lavery), Rabbi (*Zalman and the Madness of God* by E. Wiesel), and Joan of Arc (*Joan of Arc* by P. Schumann).

75.1. Subtype: Fundamentalist

Quality: More extreme than the orthodox, this type is fixed upon a dogma to the extent of becoming intolerant of other points of view. The fundamentalist is authoritarian, rigid, and self-righteous, and tends to proselytize.

Function: Fundamentalists assert the absolute truth of one belief system and attempt to impose it upon nonbelievers who are seen as infidels.

Examples: Coriolanus (*Coriolanus* by Shakespeare), Brand (*Brand* by H. Ibsen), Matthew Brady (*Inherit the Wind* by J. Lawrence and R. Lee), and Chairman Mao (*Quotations from Chairman Mao* by E. Albee).

75.2. Subtype: Ascetic (see also Pariah)

Quality: Instead of proselytizing, this austere type is reclusive, abstemious, and self-denying, a self-chosen outcast.

Function: The ascetic remains true to given philosophical and spiritual beliefs by means of removal from worldly surroundings and denial of physical and emotional distractions.

Examples: Timon (*Timon of Athens* by Shakespeare), Alceste (*The Misanthrope* by Molière), Savonarola and Silvio (*The World Is Round* by A. Salacrou), and Father Damien (*Damien* by A. Morris).

76. Role Type: Agnostic

Quality: This type of skeptic is ambivalent as to a belief in a spiritual world or god beyond that which can be experienced directly by the senses.

Function: The agnostic remains skeptical, doubting the existence of God and/or spirituality, without fully rejecting these notions.

Examples: Pentheus (*The Bacchae* by Euripides), Judas (*The Passion Play* by Anonymous), Father Fulton and Father Rawleigh (*The First Legion* by E. Lavery), Driscoll (*Bury the Dead* by I. Shaw), Martin Luther (*Luther* by J. Osborne), and Dr. Martha Livingstone (*Agnes of God* by J. Pielmeir).

77. Role Type: Atheist

Quality: The atheist is clear in the belief that God does not exist and that meaningful action can only occur through the individual.

Function: This modern type functions to deny the existence of a god and the life of the spirit, rejecting the traditional teachings and dogmas of organized religion.

Examples: Dr. Morell (*The First Legion* by E. Lavery), Paul Grosshahn (*Hinkemann* by E. Toller), Henry II (*Becket* by J. Anouilh), Goetz (*The Devil and the Good Lord* by J.-P. Sartre), Schlissel (*The Tenth Man* by P. Chayefsky), Beneatha (*A Raisin in the Sun* by L. Hansberry), Halder (*Good* by C. P. Taylor).

77.1. Subtype: Nihilist

Quality: This more extreme form of atheist is negative and cynical, rejecting not only a god, but also meaningful human action.

Function: The nihilist denies the value of all meaningful action, both human and divine.

Examples: Hummel (*The Ghost Sonata* by A. Strindberg), The Devil (*Don Juan in Hell,* play within *Man and Superman* by G. B. Shaw), Baal (*Baal* by B. Brecht), Harry Hope and Larry Slade (*The Iceman Cometh* by E. O'Neill), Nada (*State of Siege* by A. Camus), Pozzo *(Waiting for Godot* by S. Beckett), and Eddie (*Hurly Burly* by D. Rabe).

78. Role Type: Cleric

Quality: Whether priest, rabbi, nun, monk, or other spiritual leader, this moral, altruistic, selfless type is devoted to spiritual and religious matters. The cleric is also often skilled in the politics and social graces of community affairs.

Function: This type offers comfort and spiritual guidance to a congregation, and provides individuals with a model of the moral life.

Examples: Friar Lawrence (*Romeo and Juliet* by Shakespeare), Father Reder (*Professor Bernhardi* by A. Schnitzler), The Rabbi (*The Tenth Man* by P. Chayefsky), and Father Farley (*Mass Appeal* by B. Davis).

78.1. Subtype: Immoral Cleric

Quality: An alternative form of cleric is duplicitous, immoral, lecherous, and/or greedy, using his position as a means of exploiting others.

Function: This deceptive cleric functions to use the trappings of righteousness and morality as a means of satisfying selfish ends.

Examples: Sir Hugh Evans (*The Merry Wives of Windsor* by Shakespeare), Cardinal (*The Duchess of Malfi* by J. Webster), Wang (*A Man's a Man* by B. Brecht), Heinrich (*the Devil and the Good Lord* by J.-P. Sartre), and Pope Pius XII (*The Deputy* by R. Hochhuth).

78.2. Subtype: Lapsed Spiritual Leader

Quality: This type of cleric is weak, guilty, and insecure, lost between the two worlds of religion and materialism, of spirit and body.

Function: The lapsed spiritual leader wages an internal war that manifests itself in self-destructive behavior.

Examples: Pastor Manders (*Ghosts* by H. Ibsen), Shannon (*The Night of the Iguana* by T. Williams), Jacques Roux (*Marat/Sade* by P. Weiss), Father Rivard (*The Runner Stumbles* by M. Stitt), Jim Casy (*The Grapes of Wrath,* adaptation of J. Steinbeck novel by F. Galati), Reverend Johnson (*Our Country's Good* by T. Wertenbaker), and Uncle Jack (*Dancing at Lughnasa* by B. Friel).

Classification: SUPERNATURAL BEINGS

79. Role Type: God/Goddess

Quality: This rather primal theatrical type is magical, moral, and prone to influencing natural events in order to satisfy his/her godly desires.

Function: This type functions to assert power over life and death. By taking on the godly role, mortals experience a sense of transcendence.

Style: Gods and goddesses are presentational characters.

Examples: Zeus (*Prometheus Bound* by Aeschylus), Jupiter (*Amphitryon* by Plautus, *Amphitryon 38* by J. Giraudoux), God (*The Book of Job* by Anonymous), Indra's Daughter (*A Dream Play* by A. Strindberg), Venus (*One Touch of Venus* by S. J. Perelman and O. Nash), Zuss (*J. B.* by A. MacLeish), and Quetzalcotl (*La Grande Carpa de los Rasquachis* by El Teatro Campesino).

79.1. Subtype: Witty God/Goddess

Quality: One alternative type is that of the ironic, witty, and wise god/goddess.

Function: These beings offer comic relief for an audience, satirizing the limits of human and godly desires.

Style: This kind of god is equally presentational in style.

Examples: Hermes (*Plutus* by Aristophanes), Dionysus (*The Frogs* by Aristophanes), Three Gods (*The Good Woman of Setzuan* by B. Brecht), Morty/Attendant (*Steambath* by B. J. Friedman).

79.2. Subtype: Dionysian God/Goddess (see also Ecstatic One)

Quality: The quality of the Dionysian role is irrational, sexually ambivalent, orgiastic, intoxicating, and amoral.

Function: The role functions as a liberation of the human passions and spirit. In role, the Dionysian actor expresses a truly spontaneous and ecstatic nature.

Style: This is a theatre of the id and of the primal scream—one in which powerful iconoclastic images reign, conventional taboos are violated, essential passions are released, and universal truths are revealed. This fully presentational style reflects the theoretical musings of Artaud (1958), Beck (1972), and Brook (1978).

Examples: Dionysus has served as example for a number of role types described earlier: the bisexual, the trickster, the disguised one, and the ecstatic one. In *The Bacchae* by Euripedes, we meet the prototype. This androgynous Dionysus inspires his orgiastic coven of Maenads to primal acts of sex and violence. And when his power is challenged by Pentheus, the rationalist and doubter, Dionysus sexually humiliates him, then brings about his brutal murder at the hands of his mother.

The Dionysian role can be found in such characters as Shakespeare's Caliban (*The Tempest*), Brecht's Baal (*Baal*) and Macheath (*The Threepenny Opera* with K. Weill), T. Williams' Stanley Kowalski (*A Streetcar Named Desire*), P. Weiss's Marquis de Sade (*Marat/Sade*), and P. Shaffer's Alan Strang (*Equus*), to mention a few. Other characters inspired by Dionysus include Comus (*Comus* by J. Milton), Dion Anthony (*The Great God Brown* by E. O'Neill), Dr. John (*Summer and Smoke* by T. Williams), and Dionysus (*The Frogs*, adaptation of Aristophanes's play by S. Sondheim and B. Shevelove).

79.3. Subtype: Apollonian God/Godddess (see also Visionary)

Quality: In his late-19th-century analysis of Greek tragedy, Nietzsche (1872/1956) set up a dichotomy: on the one side, the ecstatic tradition of Dionysus, and on the other, the rational tradition represented by Apollo. Apollo is the embodiment of order, rationality, and beauty.

Function: The Apollonian role represents form, order, logic, grace, and poetry—a transcendence through beauty. In Greek myth and drama, Apollo is seen often as the god of prophecy, one who is consulted before a king makes a decision. To learn the source of Thebes's troubles, for example, Oedipus sends Creon to consult the oracle of Apollo. Associated with the prophetic quality, the Apollonian role becomes that of the dreamer and romantic, the magician, and the philosopher/visionary. Such qualities of Apollo serve a formal and poetic purpose.

Style: Like the Dionysian role, the Apollonian role is generally presentational in style.

Examples: In the Aeschylus play *The Eumenides*, the character Orestes, supported by the rational Apollo, stands in marked contrast to the Dionysian Furies, hounding Orestes and demanding his punishment. In *The Bacchae* by Euripides, the Apollonian figure, a foil for Dionysus is the character of Pentheus.

In the plays of Shakespeare, we find many examples of the Dionysian–Apollonian tension, including the struggle within Prince Hal and between him and his cohort, Falstaff (*Henry IV, Part II*); and that of Caliban struggling against the rational magician, Prospero (*The Tempest*).

In modern drama we find the interior struggle of the Apollonian Dr. Dysart in P. Shaffer's *Equus,* who pits his passionate fantasies against his mediocre reality. This struggle is mirrored in Dysart's encounters with his young patient, the Dionysian Alan Strang—a blinder of horses who has, in the eyes of the doctor, participated in ecstatic rites.

79.4. Subtype: Christ/Saint

Quality: The quality of the Christ role is that of the nonviolent revolutionary who loves unconditionally and exhorts others to do the same. The Christ role is one of the suffering servant, the saint and sacrificer who takes on the sins of humankind. The paradoxical form of Christ as both man and god is not unique; the Greek and Roman gods, as well as their earlier counterparts, were also depicted as such. Christ is different in his role as the messiah, the one destined to rescue humankind from its immoral tendencies.

Function: The Christ role serves, on one level, a rescuer function. On a higher level, the Christ role is a transcendent one, like the other god roles. Through assuming the role, one asserts a moral power and transcends one's spiritual vulnerabilities, participating in the unconditional love and grace of the gods.

Style: The presentational Christ role has adapted to changes in style and fashion. In his contemporary incarnations, Christ appears as both hippie clown (*Godspell* by S. Schwartz and J. M. Tebelak) and pop icon (*Jesus Christ, Superstar* by T. Rice and A. Lloyd Webber).

Examples: Other examples include Christ (*The Passion Play* by Anonymous), Eleanora (*Easter* by A. Strindberg), Violaine (*The Tidings Brought to Mary* by P. Claudel), and St. Francis of Assisi (*Clérambard* by M. Aymé).

80. Role Type: Fairy (see also Fool)

Quality: This generic type, which encompasses sprite, guardian angel, good witch, and leprechaun, is magical, delicate, innocent, endearing, romantic, and playful.

Function: Fairies amuse and delight humans, and help them solve problems.

Style: The fairy is a presentational character, well represented by Ariel in Shakespeare's *The Tempest.* This lyrical sprite conjures up storms at his master's bidding, facilitates the magic of young love, and punishes evildoers. Although he is a highly stylized character, Shakespeare endows him with a certain pathos. This sprite is a slave longing for his freedom to wander the cosmos at will.

Examples: The fairy is a mainstay of dramatic literature. Further examples include Peaseblossom (*A Midsummer Night's Dream* by Shakespeare), Rautendelein (*The Sunken Bell* by G. Hauptmann), Tinkerbell (*Peter Pan* by J. M. Barrie), Mr. Lob (*Dear Brutus* by J. M. Barrie), Ondine (*Ondine* by J. Giraudoux), The Munchkins and Glinda the Good Witch (*The Wizard of Oz* by L. F. Baum), Og (*Finian's Rainbow* by E. Y. Harburg and B. Lane), and Angels and Animals (*The Domestic Resurrection Circus* by P. Schumann).

81. Role Type: Demon (see also Beast and Deceiver)

Quality: These are the dark inhabitants of the spirit world: Furies, Maenads, witches, and ghosts, who are magical and evil, threatening and powerful.

Function: Demons add the dimension of fear and dread to the world of human experience, saving humankind from complacency and self-righteousness.

Style: Demonic role types are portrayed presentationally.

Examples: The Furies (*The Bacchae* by Euripides), The Three Witches (*Macbeth* by Shakespeare), Mummy (*The Ghost Sonata* by A. Strindberg), The Flies (*The Flies* by J. -P. Sartre), John (*Dark of the Moon* by H. Richardson and W. Barney), Dracula (*Dracula: Sabbat* by L. Katz), and Witch (*Into the Woods* by J. Lapine and S. Sondheim).

81.1. Subtype: Satan

Quality: This classic devil is the tempter, a fallen angel, the antithesis of Christ and God; he is the primary symbol of evil in the Judeo-Christian tradition.

Function: The Satanic function is to oppose righteousness and godliness, and to tempt humans to choose evil over good.

Style: Satan, like other demons, is a presentational figure.

Examples: Mephistopheles, the demonic tempter of Faust, first created in theatre by Marlowe in *Doctor Faustus,* is threatening and powerful, capable of negotiating the ultimate fate of human souls. Like other Satanic characters, he is the personification of evil, a type that continues to appeal to audiences in the many popular horror movies concerning possession and supernatural threat.

The endless array of Satanic characters includes the following: Satan (*The Book of Job* by Anonymous), Mephistopheles (*Faust* by J. W. von Goethe), The Devil and Dickon (*The Scarecrow* by P. MacKaye), The Magician (*The Wonder-Working Magician* by P. Calderon), Nickles (*J. B.* by A. MacLeish), Mr. Applegate (*Damn Yankees* by G. Abbott, D. Wallop, and F. Loesser), and The Serpent (*The Serpent* by J. -C. van Itallie).

81.2. Subtype: Death

Quality: Death is one of the earliest roles personified in ancient dramatic rituals. As a type, death is threatening and terrifying, the incarnation of nonbeing.

Function: This type functions to claim the lives of mortals.

Style: Death appears in presentational style.

Examples: The white-faced character of Death that appears in Ingmar Bergman's highly theatrical film *The Seventh Seal*, set during the Middle Ages, is an excellent rendering of this role type, familiar to most cultures in various ritual forms. Examples of this ubiquitous character in theatre history include Death (*Everyman* by Anonymous), Death (*Orpheus* by J. Cocteau), Death (*On Borrowed Time* by P. Osborn), Death (*State of Siege* by A. Camus), and Death (*Totentanz* by P. Schumann).

82. Role Type: Magician

Quality: The magician, also encompassing the sorcerer/sorceress, is powerful in the ability to transform the natural world. This type is in control of supernatural forces, which can be summoned to serve good or evil purposes.

Function: The magician uses supernatural powers to alter the course of natural events.

Style: This type is generally presented in a stylized fashion.

Example: Shakespeare offers an example of the magician in the character of Prospero in *The Tempest.* Prospero's tempest is stirred up in order to punish his deceptive and usurping brother. In the bargain, the further magic of love and forgiveness occurs; all is righted with the world, and the aging magician retires his magic.

The role of magician has become not only that of an individual character among others, but an act, usually within variety or burlesque shows, in its own right. Harry Houdini popularized the one-person magic show in the early part of the 20th century. Contemporary magicians, such as Penn and Teller, have revived that tradition, adding certain postmodern touches.

Examples of classical and modern magicians include Oberon and Titania (*A Midsummer Night's Dream* by Shakespeare), John Wellinton Wells (*The Sorcerer* by W. S. Gilbert and A. Sullivan), the Conjurer (*Magic* by G. K. Chesterton), The Stage Manager (*Our Town* by T. Wilder), and The Player King (*Rosencrantz and Guildenstern Are Dead* by T. Stoppard).

DOMAIN: AESTHETIC

83. Role Type: Artist

Quality: Ibsen's depictions of the architect Solness (*The Master Builder*) and the artist Rubek (*When We Dead Awaken*) represent early studies of the artist as tormented, a modern version of this role type. The artist as type is sensitive, creative, isolated, and often long-suffering.

Function: The role type functions to assert the creative principle, envisioning new forms and transforming old ones. Because of the spiritual demands and responsibilities of the aesthetic process, the artist often pays an emotional price. In many ways, the modern artist becomes an ambivalent person, unsure of the value of his art and of the boundaries between art and life.

Examples: Aeschylus and Euripides (*The Frogs* by Aristophanes), Manrico (*The Troubadour* by A. Garcia Gutierrez), Dubedat (*The Doctor's Dilemma* by G. B. Shaw), Von Sala (*The Lonely Way* by A. Schnitzler), Dearth (*Dear Brutus* by J. M. Barrie), Orpheus (*Legend of Lovers* by J. Anouilh), and George (*Sunday in the Park with George* by J. Lapine and S. Sondheim).

83.1. Subtype: Performer (see also Beauty and Narcissist)

Quality: The artist frequently appears in drama as actor. This performing artist is mask-like, distancing, egocentric, and extroverted, eager to please and to be applauded.

Function: The performer seeks to be accepted and praised by an audience for his performance.

Examples: Bottom (*A Midsummer Night's Dream* by Shakespeare), The Player King (*Hamlet* by Shakespeare), Kean (*Kean* by J.-P Sartre), Archie Rice (*The Entertainer* by J. Osborne), Kaspar (*Kaspar* by P. Handke), Robert and John (*A Life in the Theatre* by D. Mamet), and Sir John (*The Dresser* by R. Harwood).

84. Role Type: Dreamer

Quality: The dreamer is an idealist and romantic, living in a self-made fantasy world.

Function: This type fantasizes about a more desirable existence and remains aloof from the world of the present.

Style: The dreamer is generally a stylized, romantic character.

Examples: Romeo (*Romeo and Juliet* by Shakespeare), Treplev

(*The Sea Gull* by A. Chekhov), Robert Mayo (*Beyond the Horizon* by E. O'Neill), The Young Dreamer (*Within the Gates* by S. O'Casey), Don Quixote (*Man of La Mancha,* by D. Wasserman, M. Leigh, and J. Darion), and Max, Arthur, and Nancy (*The Goodbye People* by H. Gardner).

THE USE AND SIGNIFICANCE OF THE TAXONOMY

From playing god to playing sign, the actor and the role have endured throughout the millennia. Even as the times have radically changed, the types of theatrical roles played by actors have remained remarkably constant.

Although the taxonomy presents a listing of 84 independent types, role types do not exist in a vacuum. Each Antigone has her Creon, each Juliet her Romeo, each Estragon his Vladimir. If any one character is removed from a play, the entire structure will then change. Remove Ophelia from *Hamlet,* for example, and the sexual, romantic theme is lost. The hero moves in a dramatic world of deceivers, villains, and helpers. Fools subsist with simpletons and wise people. Victims exist in a dramatic world of victimizers and survivors. Thus the notion of interactive and interrelated roles is implicit within the taxonomy.

A dramatic world as represented by its characters is a fragile structure that does not easily admit tinkering. As constructed by a playwright, each role has a defined status and function. Relationships are carefully developed for dramatic purposes, often in the service of the hero.

The dramatic world of a play is a planned one, a constructed artifice in which characters are clearly established by given lines, actions, and motivations. When that world is so well constructed that it presents certain essential truths, it does so in the guise of characters or roles. In extending the metaphor of people as players, the dramatic world of a play has a psychological counterpart in the role system—an interior cast of characters that provides structure and coherence to an individual's everyday existence. The role system is not planned by a godlike playwright, but is constructed over a lifetime of experiences in roles that are inherited, taken on from the social world, and played out behaviorally.

The taxonomy represents an attempt to identify those essential role types that have appeared and reappeared in some of the most prominent plays within Western dramatic literature. In placing the role types within a context of quality, function, and style, a dramatic model emerges that applies to the use of role not only in theatre, but also in everyday life and drama therapy—where role can provide a way of viewing the mysteries of life lived dialectically, in and out of the looking glass.

As applied to everyday life, the taxonomy offers a glimpse into the role system, a view of the personae that may provide the essential elements of the personality. As a dramatic model, the taxonomy is one way of conceptualizing behavior and motivation. With the taxonomy as a map, individuals may be better able to understand their various journeys. In retrospect, the meaning of my journey to Mount Athos became clearer as I was able to identify the role conflicts encountered in that strange land and to understand how the invoked roles served me there and continue to serve me in my everyday life.

As we have seen in Chapters Four through Six, theatrical role types can also inform the process of healing through drama. Michael and Ann, for example, were able to name and transform various internal roles that seemed to control too much of their behavior. With the availability of the taxonomy, both therapist and client may approach the healing process with a clearer sense of the qualities, functions, and styles of such roles as victim and hero. With that knowledge, the players in the therapeutic drama can better identify the essential roles to be explored and move toward a more appropriate means of enacting them.

One major component of this book has been its stories, beginning with a personal one of a spiritual journey. Personal stories have been complemented by literary and therapeutic ones. Each story— whether fictional or not, whether generated for theatrical, therapeutic, or everyday purposes—can be understood, at one level, in terms of its characters. The taxonomy offers a systematic view not of specific characters in stories, but of character or role types that seem to embody archetypal qualities. In applying the taxonomy to an analysis of dramatic, therapeutic, or everyday stories, one is able to make sense of the storyteller, if not of the story. For one reason people may seek out and generate stories is to find themselves therein. The taxonomy can serve as a guide for all on that search.

On the one hand, then, the taxonomy is an abstraction, a picture of the role system in terms of the content, function, and style of its individual parts. On the other hand, the taxonomy can serve a utilitarian purpose, as a map for drama therapists and others to find their way and to make sense of their presentations in role.

CHAPTER TWELVE

Conclusion

Know thyself.
—SOCRATES

Know your customers.
—UNCLE HARRY

Folk wisdom, in one version from the mouth of my Uncle Harry, informs us: "Know your customers." For my Uncle Harry, that knowledge came in handy when he was trying to sell an extra pair of pants to a reluctant buyer. For me, it implies more than just commerce. If I know my customers, I can not only sell them my wares, but also know who I am when in their presence. They are, in Mead's (1934) terminology, the "generalized other" —the social group that I must internalize in order to know how to play out my complementary role.

In the presence of a significant social group, I en-role. The more I know their expectations of me and mine of them, the more likely I will be to play out a functional version of the role. If I need to sell a suit of clothes, I will play out my salesman role based upon a knowledge of how well the customer trusts me, what his needs are, and how much I can expect him to spend.

When I am completely out of my element, among unknown customers who speak a foreign language, I tend either to become fearful and overly cautious or to retreat to older roles, hoping that they will somehow get me through. On Mount Athos, in the face of threatening ascetics and tricksters, I went through a series of roles—coward and victim, ambivalent one and moralist—until I could find those familiar "customers" who would engage me in more familiar ways, drawing out more comfortable roles. In the company of a helper, I began to feel safer. In relation to an orthodox believer and a skeptical libertine, I knew I was on familiar territory, as these men invoked corresponding parts of my own psyche.

A colleague, whom I had known as a witty person, was visiting his daughter, who worked as an English teacher in a foreign culture many thousands of miles from home. Being a New Yorker who had been mugged in the city once before, he felt generally cautious about walking around unfamiliar streets. One day he found himself alone and lost while touring the foreign city. It was getting late, and he realized that he could neither read a street sign nor find any friendly person who spoke English. Each time he turned a corner, he felt more lost. Each time he reached out to an individual on the street, he was rebuffed and felt humiliated. He became aware of how different he looked from the others, and began to notice the stares of passers-by. A woman and her young daughter approached him directly, too close for his comfort. The woman thrust her finger aggressively toward his face and spoke in an agitated manner to her daughter. Retreating to a familiar role of victim, my friend found himself giving up control and expecting to be hurt or at least humiliated. Yet he countered the woman's gesture by smiling broadly and responding in loud, insistent tones: "Hello, how are you?" They looked at him as if he were mad, then eventually left, leaving him to fend for himself.

He stopped for a moment, caught his breath, and realized that he was unharmed and that his daughter could not be too far away. With the help of a map and a sympathetic non-English-speaking street vendor who was amused by his foolishness, he was able to navigate the winding streets and locate the road back to his daughter's house. He was a survivor after all.

Had he better understood the cultural milieu, he might have avoided the plunge into the victim role. Yet once there, he smiled as if to say: "I'm a nice person. Don't hurt me." And thus far, despite a random attack on the streets of New York, he has managed to get through life relatively unscathed, transforming the victim part of himself to the survivor.

This story recalls Ann's moments in the kitchen with her inebriated father (see Chapter Six). He was dangerous and potentially violent as he sharpened his knife. And she, desperately afraid of slipping into the victim role, joked him out of his role as victimizer.

Bruno Bettelheim (*The Empty Fortress*, 1967) writes about the role that concentration camp victims during World War II needed to take on in order to survive the daily horrors. Many became zombies, shutting down feeling, refusing to see the atrocities right before their eyes.

Bettelheim compares this condition to that of autism and schizophrenia, in which the individual shuts off all communication with the outside world, which is seen as terrifying and brutal. Reports of survivors of the brutalities of the killing fields of Cambodia, where the Khmer Rouge committed unspeakable atrocities (see Cooke, 1991), state that a high percentage of refugee Cambodian women who have settled in southern California have become blind with no apparent physiological explanation. (This situation has led playwright Ernest Abuba to create a musical theatre piece, *Cambodia Agonistes*, which premiered at the Pan-Asian Repertory Playhouse in New York City in 1992.)

Those who are able to transform their role of victim to that of survivor know their customers. They choose the role qualities that will get them through, whether a foolish grin, a deadened affect, or a blindness. As fool or zombie, they are able to survive the terror.

Victims of psychological abuse also become survivors by virtue of finding a way to defuse the terror of their victimizers. Michael and Ann did it through therapy, slowly working through the fear of their fathers, whom they perceived as wielding an axe and a knife, ready to cut down the sexual and intimate needs of their children. The therapeutic process helped them invoke not only their dreaded fathers (and mothers), but also the murderous, rageful parts of themselves that blocked their ability to seek out functional adult relationships.

Knowing your customers is one part of the folk wisdom. Another part is finding an appropriate response in role, to allow you to survive well in the presence of the customer. And yet a third missing part, I would now tell my Uncle Harry, is knowing your stock. If a man is short and I only have long coats on the rack, I cannot sell him a coat, given the moral quality that I attach to my salesman role. But if my stock is varied—if I have a variety of sizes and styles—I will make the sale.

My Uncle Harry, like many members of the generation that came of age during the Great Depression, saw things in basic moral tones, blacks and whites. You either sold a suit of clothes or you didn't. You either had a buck in your pocket or you were broke. His life style, like that of Sam (the compulsive accountant referred to in Chapter Two), was greatly limited. Although a survivor of the depressions and wars, as Harry grew older he felt more and more like a victim. The times changed; the liberation movements of women, young people, and blacks exploded around him. The family became a further source of indignity as nieces and nephews asserted their needs for liberation from the old ways.

Harry was unambivalent to the end. He knew his customers and he knew his stock. But with the inevitable changes of fashion, this unambivalent man was left with few customers, a depleted stock, and a limited role system. He died a bitter man, having allowed the role of survivor to slip into that of victim. The victim role served him well to the end, perpetuating his feelings of abandonment, isolation, and rage.

Many, like Harry, strive to live the unambivalent life alone. But the price is very high indeed. Others, with similar aims, join apparently safe collectives represented by religious cults, political ideologies, or corporations, offering their loyalty and allegiance in exchange for the security of lives with clear, unambiguous rules and boundaries. In doing so, however, they abrogate some of the role complexity that comes only from struggling through choices. A life lived in isolation or in the bosom of a self-contained collective is an unheroic life. Martin Buber, the wise philosopher who wrote of the need for effective human communication (see *Between Man and Man,* 1948), referred to both extremes—the egocentric and the collectivistic—as antithetical to the life of dialogue, a state of open exchange between people.

To live the life of dialogue, an ability to engage with another responsibly, one must allow ambivalence in. Ambivalence is a state of uncertainty as to who one is, where one is going, and why one needs to go there. In dialogue—not only an open exchange between people, but also a reasoning through one's inner voices—one begins to work through the uncertainties and to become aware of options. Ambivalence implies choice, and choice implies the possibility of alternative thought and action. In dialogue with another, there is the possibility that one's point of view will be challenged and that one will need to take on the voice of the other in order to advance this point of view. The life of dialogue requires an open role system since one engages in dialogue through role, each role representing a specific point of view.

In specifying a taxonomy of roles, it is my intention to systematically lay out many of the role choices one can make. As previously mentioned, it is not clear just how much choice one has, as primary roles appear to be given and secondary roles appear to be taken on from the social world, for the most part unconsciously. Yet even when they are biologically or socially determined, roles are subject to modification in terms of quality, function, and style. Furthermore, roles tend to be transformed as an individual experiences a change in consciousness, relationship, status, or stature. This has been seen in the case of Michael, for example, when he experienced a movement from victim to victor in the process of drama therapy.

In many ways, the dramatic role method offers a natural solution to the many dilemmas that need to be addressed throughout life. For example, one of the early potential traumas confronted by a young child is the change in status from only child to older child who must suddenly share the love of the parents with a newborn sibling. As an only child, my daughter, Georgie, thoroughly enjoyed all the privileges of her status, receiving unconditional love and attention from her mother and me. As an exclusively breast-fed child for the first 6 months of her life, she luxuriated in the ethos of feeding on demand. When she was 18 months old, however, her world changed radically: A brother was born, and with him the ambivalences set in. Suddenly she had to construct a completely new role—that of big sister. Suddenly she had to reconstruct her role as daughter and find a new way to internalize the role of parents. All at once, she no longer knew her customers.

When Georgie first arrived at the hospital to greet the cause of all her ambivalence, the baby was absent. Her mother and I had planned to allow her to remain in role for a while longer. Her mother gave her a present, a large stuffed dog, and welcomed her warmly after a long day and a half of separation. She would have none of it. She knew that something was up and that she was about to be dethroned. As a consequence, she refused to interact with her mother at all.

I took Georgie with me to retrieve the baby from the nursery, and together we wheeled him back to her mother's room. She was allowed to hold the baby and begin to try out her new role as big sister. But then it was time to nurse, and at the sight of the new baby on her mother's breast, Georgie became distraught, crying: "No! That's Daddy's baby. No, no!" The potential loss of her mother was very hurtful.

Her mother offered Georgie the other breast as she nursed the newborn. In doing so, she allowed her to regress a bit—to stay with the old secure role of daughter and baby, unconditionally lovable, ready to be nourished at any time. She went for the breast briefly, then allowed herself to return to her present dilemma: to be Mama's favored, unconditionally lovable child or not to be.

During the next several weeks, Georgie struggled with her role ambivalence of daughter versus orphan, only child versus big sister, loved one versus rejected one. A resolution seemed to occur one day when I read her "Peter Rabbit." In the story, Peter, one of four siblings, disobeys his mother and gets into trouble. In search of good food, he trespasses in the garden of a mean farmer. Peter is discovered and is chased so far that he gets lost in the unfamiliar terrain. He finally makes it home and is reunited with his siblings and his mother, who fixes him chamomile tea and tucks him safely into bed.

During the reading, Georgie became fixated upon the page illustrating Peter as lost. She would cry out in a half-serious, half-ironic tone: "Ooh, he got lost!" Each time I read the story, she would insist that I return to the lost Peter page. Then she would flip forward to the image of the mother offering him tea, with Peter lying safely in bed, noting in a relieved tone: "Ohh, his Mommy . . . Peter safe. Oh, Mommy."

Within 8 weeks of losing her status as only child, Georgie partially worked through her anxiety. Like Peter, she had felt lost and abandoned, tossed out by her mother into hostile territory to fend for herself. Through the fictional story, she relived her fears many times over, engaging in the process that Freud aptly named the "repetition compulsion."

But in order to move beyond the lost daughter, she had to build upon the role of big sister. She worked diligently at this, demanding to participate in the rituals of nurturing her brother. She assisted in his diapering and his feeding. When the baby cried, her mother asked: "What should I do?" and Georgie responded: "Put Mama's breast." When her mother and I weren't around, she offered the crying baby the pacifier, a substitute breast. As she experienced these activities, Georgie was also beginning to take on the mother role. This culminated with a request to nurse the baby on her own breast within a week of her second birthday.

She was further allowed to regress from time to time and to take on some of the privileges of the baby—lying in his carriage (which was once her carriage), being diapered on his changing table (which was once her table), being held on demand.

The story of Peter Rabbit helped model the way home—the return from the role of the lost one to the lovable daughter, reunited with her sibling and mother. As such, the story provided a natural means of healing through role.

The role method is indicated in treatment when the natural means of identification and working through role becomes impaired, leading a person to become stuck at the level of the repetition compulsion. The role method, like any other therapeutic process, is limited to those willing and ready to take their heroic journeys toward discovery. For extreme isolates and ideologues, therapy is for the most part futile. The therapeutic process can only proceed if persons are able to experience ambivalence within the single role at the cornerstone of their belief system, or between opposing roles.

Role ambivalence is essential for growth and change, whether in everyday life or in therapy. When it is too overwhelming, some form of help is needed to restore a modicum of balance. But when it causes a level of imbalance that challenges one to search for a solution to a particular dilemma, then it will indeed lead to healthy development.

As mentioned earlier, role ambivalence occurs at three levels: within a role as opposing qualities conflict, between opposing roles, and as an existential state of being and nonbeing. The first two are rather straightforward in terms of understanding both the natural process of healing through role (as in the example of Georgie) and an applied process of healing (as in the cases of Michael and Ann). In working through their role ambivalences, these individuals were able to discover ways of solving problems and creating more functional role systems.

The third level of role ambivalence is more basic and more difficult to conceptualize. It embodies a central thesis of this book: that role concerns a movement in and out of given states of being, and that in order to develop fully, people need to discover ways to live in and among their roles no matter how deeply they conflict. Hamlet's dilemma, as such, needs to be revised from a choice between life and death to a state that allows both aspects to coexist within a single role system. In order to survive within a threatening environment (both inside and out), one needs first to acknowledge the existence of the fearful parts, and then to discover ways to live with them. Like Athena in *The Eumenides*, who appeases the angry Furies by allowing them an honored place in Athenian society, we too need to allow space for our psychological terrors; if they are denied, they will certainly not rest until they have overrun our role systems.

The image of Hamlet has run throughout this book because I see him as the prototypical ambivalent one who sets up the ultimate choice between the forces of life and death. As one of the most frequently produced plays in history, *Hamlet* galvanizes many of the concerns of its audiences. Like Hamlet, we too become confused when in the presence of a seductive mother, a victimized father, a murderous stepfather, a suicidal lover, traitorous and fawning friends, and spying elders. We too wrestle with our ambivalent thoughts concerning the legitimacy, love, and fidelity of these seeming intimates. We too struggle with our feelings of chaste and sexual love, vengeance and forgiveness, connection and betrayal, self-love and self-hate, wisdom and ignorance, action and passivity. And, like Hamlet, we wonder whether we can really trust our visions.

Hamlet's method of seeking the truth of his existential dilemma is an indirect one. Like Hamlet, we often mask our real feelings and take on social personae as we attempt "through indirection to search direction out." Such is the role method—an indirect approach to healing, requiring the distance and safety afforded by a persona, a mask, a role. Hamlet plays the fool, one of diminished status but superior intelligence, in order to probe and test those whom he loves and hates. But this is no ordinary fool; Hamlet's version is heroic in stature, tragic in consequence. This fool is a mask of the hero.

We may choose any number of roles that serve to uncover the mysteries we need to solve. Like Georgie, we may choose Peter Rabbit; like Michael, the boy who learned to burn; like Ann, Hansel; or like Julia, the evil mother. These roles, too, may be masks of the hero to the extent that we take them on to further a psychological and often mysterious journey. The Hamlet within us is heroic and searching, driven by ambivalence, accepting of the dark roles that will inevitably surface along the way, and committed to struggling with the contradictions of existence.

As stated above, one possible reading of *Hamlet* is that all characters, including Hamlet's own subroles, subsist as projections of the Prince of Denmark. Thus, Gertrude may represent the mother part of Hamlet; Ophelia, the lover–sister part; the ghost and Claudius, the father part; Horatio, the loyal friend part; Rosencrantz and Guildenstern, the betrayer parts; Polonius, the simpleton part; Laertes, the brother part; Fortinbras, the victor part; the Players, the performer part; and so on. When interrelated, these and other roles (e.g., sentinels, messengers, and fools) comprise a personality. Such a reading is close to the spirit of this book in its insistence upon the one as many, the personality as a system of persona.

Hamlet is Everyman and Everywoman, with many and various roles intact even as they conflict. And at the same time Hamlet is no man or woman, but simply a fiction, some wonderful words on a piece of paper. As everyday actors we can, with some effort, read our own lives as a story. In fact, when telling stories about our experiences, we often tend to see ourselves as our favorite characters—Hamlet, Peter Rabbit, Hansel, or Gretel, for example. And then we step back, no longer in any discernible role, and wonder: Is this the person that I am? Is this the way I want it to be? The answer will ultimately lead back to the roles. I am that which I continue to reveal through behavior in role. And I am that which I conceal through thoughts and feelings embodied in unexplored and unacknowledged roles. I am like my mother in some ways and different from her in others. I am a friend to some and a betrayer to others. I am all of these things and many more to myself. If I can contain these roles well in the wide net that is my personality, I can truly learn to live in the ambivalence that appears to hold the roles in balance.

In the absence of a god, individuals invent other gods. In the absence of a self, we tend to invent systems that address such basic questions as: Who am I? The role system offers one response: I am a creator and creation of my roles, which taken together provide coherence to my life, even as they interrelate in a paradoxical fashion. The taxonomy of roles is one way of specifying the contents of the role system.

My primary source for conceptualizing the role system is that of theatre, which may in itself be limited to certain repeated types, most of which were conceived in the classical Greek and Roman theatre. In concluding my research, I feel that the spectrum of roles offered in theatre is fairly comprehensive as it relates to everyday behavior. Whenever a new role type is discovered, however, in everyday life or in drama therapy or in other dramatic forms, the taxonomy will need to expand. A new role will be one with discernible qualities, functions, and style. If the role is not derived from theatre, then clinical and/or everyday sources will need to be specified to justify its inclusion within the taxonomy of roles.

In my years of working in the performance, educational, and therapeutic modes of drama, I have never quite been able to pinpoint the essential "selfness" or core of the art form. Could it be that all characters and knowledge and healing that spring from drama are ultimately paradoxical? Could it be that drama can never be seen as one thing because it exists in the space between being and nonbeing, between en-roling and de-roling, between the enhanced life and the ordinary one, between the spiritual voyage and the road back home? It seems clear to me that without ambivalence there can be no drama. A character onstage, in a script, or in an applied dramatic improvisation is, by definition, suspended between two realities: the one of the role and the other of the actor portraying the role. And within the context of the drama, the character generally confronts opposing voices—either internally, as in soliloquy, or externally, as in the conflict between hero and villain.

In extending the *theatricum mundi* metaphor, I further propose that without ambivalence there can be no movement or growth in everyday life. The two certain ways of denying ambivalence, as mentioned above, are taking on the role of the isolate or taking on the role of the ideologue. The former is represented in the taxonomy as the lost one; the latter is represented as the fundamentalist. In both instances, individuals assume extreme positions as a means of silencing the voices of contradiction. Those belonging to a diminutive society of ascetics (such as the hermits on Mount Athos), or the followers of such expansive organizations as the Jehovah's Witnesses, choose to live a life of limited roles, trusting in more spiritual rewards further down the line. Within their world views, their choices are well justified, and many are able to function well within their chosen cultures and ideologies. But yet, even as the body abstains, even as the conscious mind restricts itself to extreme forms of discipline and denial, the role system still manufactures dreams, fantasies, and contrary visions, no matter how small.

Perhaps at the very center of the dramatic world view is the question often attributed to Stanislavsky in his role as actor trainer: "What if?" For Ann, like Hamlet, a version of that question became: "What if I killed my father?" For Michael, the question took many forms: "What if I let go of my rage? What if I let myself trust another man? What if I took the AIDS test? What if I am lovable and allow myself to love another person?" The connection among the three parts of this book—everyday life, drama, and therapy—can be made through the question "What if?" It marks a readiness to move from things as they are to things as they might be. It opens up the potentiality of being something other than a self, a single thing that is fixed and good. It leads one away from that which is already known and safe into the less predictable realm of possibility. It is a bridge connecting the ordinary and the extraordinary. It is the question that provokes enhanced dramatic moments in everyday life and persuades one to take risks. It is the stuff that motivates scientific research and artistic creation. It is, essentially, a question about role. In asking, "What if I kill my father?", I contemplate taking on the role of murderer or rebel or avenger or liberator. And as the question is posed, an ambivalence sets in: What will be the consequences of my action in role? Can I live with the guilt? What if I turn the weapon on myself and end all the anguish . . . or do not act at all?

Hamlet answers his own existential questions with a simple statement: "Readiness is all." When one is ready to accept the contradictory pulls and often painful role confusions, then one will act. Killing a father is a relatively easy act once one is ready to pull the trigger.

The connections among drama, everyday life, and therapy can be discovered on many levels. Throughout this book, I have attempted to link the three by means of the concept of role and a dramatic model of role analysis, specifying role types and their qualities, functions, and styles. The work that remains is to push the model a step further into a full-blown theory of role—one that can generate significant research questions for drama therapists and others looking for ways of making sense of the ordinary and extraordinary drama of existence.

I would like to conclude with an anecdote. Some years ago I had a friend, Will, who seemed conflicted in terms of his roles. He was an athletic man who took great pride in his physical competence and competitiveness. He worked hard in college and law school. When he graduated, he was idealistic and attempted to become a civil rights lawyer, protecting the disenfranchised. But he couldn't get a job in the prestigious civil rights firms. After some soul-searching, he recognized that he really wanted to make a lot of money and vowed to become the most successful collections lawyer in his area. He did not consciously recognize the dilution of his ideals.

In his former quest for socially meaningful work, he dressed and identified with the hippie lifestyle, as he understood it. In his latter quest, he traded in his turtlenecks and bellbottoms for three-piece suits and became a bona fide yuppie. In fact, for a period of several years, his politics and lifestyle changed as frequently as the current fashions.

I had not seen Will in 25 years. Upon our reunion, he appeared softer, less cocky, and less fashionable. He was now a trial lawyer, diversified and content in his professional and family life. He told me a story:

Some years ago, after achieving financial success in his law practice, he ventured out into a business deal, opening up a fast-food franchise with a partner. It seemed a sure thing. He found that he didn't have the time or energy to attend to the business, so he hired his father to manage it. His father was retired; a widower, he had recently remarried and was living well beyond his means. Throughout the year he would ask his son for "loans," and Will would feel obliged to write out checks for the man who was once a pillar of strength to him, who had put him through college and law school.

As the months passed, his father asked Will for more and more money. As he wrote out the checks, Will experienced a feeling of resentment in the pit of his stomach. Within a short time, Will and his partner became alarmed: Bills were unpaid, employees were unhappy, and customers became scarce. When they examined the books, it became clear that the place was mismanaged and that Will's father was skimming off more than his share of the dwindling profits.

Will tried to turn his back on this state of affairs, but found himself again writing exorbitant checks each month to cover his father's losses. As things got to the breaking point, Will confronted his father with the books. He had finally dared to ask himself the dreaded question: "What if I fired my father?"

Caught up in his ambivalence, Will lived in a state of anxiety for a number of years. He fancied himself a good and loving son, and attempted to support his father as his father had supported him. As he grew older, Will would look in the mirror and see a reflection of his father—a man he had always seen as strong, tall, competent, wealthy, and wise. His search for an appropriate professional role was in many ways an attempt to equal his father's competence. Always falling short, Will saw himself as a lost one, a mannequin in search of the right suit of clothes to dress up his spiritual nakedness.

In going through a role reversal with his father, Will came face to face with a truth that he was finally ready to see: His father was imperfect. He had grown old and needy, losing much of his former power. He was no longer a godlike pillar of strength, and Will was no longer a worshiper at his feet. He was now a grown-up, a successful lawyer whose job was to argue a case based upon the truth of empirical evidence. In the case of his father, the facts were all in the books. In recognizing his guilt, Will was ready to rise above his own guilt and fire his father.

In symbolically killing the king, Will was finally able to dismiss the false qualities of father he had carried around all his life. In truth, Will now saw this man as a fallible human being wrestling with his own inadequacies and deserving, if not of Will's money, then at least of his compassion. In recognizing this, Will was ready to let go of his need to be the most fashionable, successful, and powerful man in the land. He too could be fallible and weak, even as he struggled to live a meaningful, successful existence.

Indeed, "The Child is father of the Man," as Wordsworth (1807/1965) has suggested. The ambivalence of being implies an existence based in struggle between conflicting roles. On the other side of the struggle is not resolution, but transformation. In this book, we have seen a number of examples of sons and daughters attempting to move beyond the control of fathers who wielded a terrible and confusing power. In staying with the journey, they recognized the need ultimately to find more positive ways to father themselves. Their symbolic murder of the father implied a transformation of the father role from victimizer to protector, from angry, needy child to intact adult, capable of meeting life's ambivalences head on.

Without the struggle between conflicting roles, there would be no drama. The undramatic life is a fool's (simpleton's) paradise. The dramatic life is one lived in paradox. And to live dramatically, one must cultivate a role system flexible enough to support and contain the struggle.

The Taxonomy of Roles
(Short Version)

DOMAIN: SOMATIC

Classification: AGE

1. Role Type: Child
2. Role Type: Adolescent
3. Role Type: Adult
4. Role Type: Elder (*see also* Grandparent)
4.1. Subtype: Lecher

Classification: SEXUAL ORIENTATION

5. Role Type: Eunuch
6. Role Type: Homosexual
7. Role Type: Transvestite
8. Role Type: Bisexual

Classification: APPEARANCE

9. Role Type: Beauty (*see also* Innocent and Immoralist)
9.1. Subtype: Seductress/Seducer
10. Role Type: Beast (*see also* Physically Disabled and Demon)
10.1. Subtype: Innocent Beast
11. Role Type: Average One (*see also* Middle Class, Lost One, Everyman, and Antihero)

Classification: HEALTH

12. Role Type: Mentally Ill/Mad Person
13. Role Type: Physically Disabled or Deformed (*see also* Beast)
13.1. Subtype: Deformed as Transcendent

14.   Role Type: Hypochondriac
15.   Role Type: Doctor
15.1. Subtype: Quack Doctor

DOMAIN: COGNITIVE

16.   Role Type: Simpleton
16.1. Subtype: Cuckold
17.   Role Type: Fool
17.1. Subtype: Trickster (*see also* Fairy)
17.2. Subtype: Existential Clown
18.   Role Type: Ambivalent One
18.1. Subtype: Disguised One
18.2. Subtype: Double
19.   Role Type: Critic
20.   Role Type: Wise Person (*see also* Visionary)
20.1. Subtype: Intellectual
20.2. Subtype: PseudoIntellectual/Pedant

DOMAIN: AFFECTIVE

Classification: MORAL

21.   Role Type: Innocent (*see also* Child and Beauty)
22.   Role Type: Villain
23.   Role Type: Deceiver (*see also* Beast, Immoralist, and Demon)
24.   Role Type: Moralist (*see also* Innocent)
24.1. Subtype: Hypocritical Moralist
24.2. Subtype: Idealist
25.   Role Type: Immoralist
25.1. Subtype: Libertine
25.2. Subtype: Adulterer/Adulteress
26.   Role Type: Victim
26.1. Subtype: Martyr
26.2. Subtype: Self-Serving Martyr
27.   Role Type: Opportunist
28.   Role Type: Bigot
29.   Role Type: Avenger
30.   Role Type: Helper
31.   Role Type: Philistine
32.   Role Type: Miser
33.   Role Type: Coward
33.1. Subtype: Braggart/Braggart Warrior (*see also* Narcissist)
34.   Role Type: Parasite
35.   Role Type: Survivor

Classification: FEELING STATES

36.   Role Type: Zombie

36.1. Subtype: Lost One (*see also* Pariah)

37.   Role Type: Malcontent

37.1. Subtype: Cynic

37.2. Subtype: Hothead

37.3. Subtype: Shrew

37.4. Subtype: Rebel

38.   Role Type: Lover

38.1. Subtype: Narcissist/Egotist (*see also* Braggart)

39.   Role Type: Ecstatic One (*see also* Dionysian God/Goddess)

DOMAIN: SOCIAL

Classification: FAMILY

40.   Role Type: Mother

40.1. Subtype: Murderous Mother

40.2. Subtype: Revolutionary Mother

41.   Role Type: Wife

41.1. Subtype: Liberated Wife

41.2. Subtype: Castrating Wife

42.   Role Type: Mother-in-law

43.   Role Type: Widow/Widower

44.   Role Type: Father

44.1. Subtype: Tyrannical Father

45.   Role Type: Husband

45.1. Subtype: Brutal Husband

45.2. Subtype: Weak Husband

46.   Role Type: Son

46.1. Subtype: Renegade/Rebel Son

46.2. Subtype: Bastard Son/Prodigal Son

47.   Role Type: Daughter

47.1. Subtype: Renegade/Rebel Daughter

47.2. Subtype: Bastard Daughter/Vengeful Daughter

47.3. Subtype: Daughter in Distress/Daughter as Victim

48.   Role Type: Sister

48.1. Subtype: Renegade/Rebel Sister

49.   Role Type: Brother

49.1. Subtype: Renegade/Rebel Brother

50.   Role Type: Grandparent (*see also* Elder)

50.1. Subtype: Senile or Mad Old Person

Classification: POLITICS/GOVERNMENT

51.   Role Type: Reactionary
52.   Role Type: Conservative
52.1. Subtype: Traditionalist
53.   Role Type: Pacifist
54.   Role Type: Revolutionary
54.1. Subtype: Self-Serving Revolutionary
55.   Role Type: Head of State
56.   Role Type: Minister/Advisor/Councillor
56.1. Subtype: Moral Minister
57.   Role Type: Bureaucrat

Classification: LEGAL

58.   Role Type: Lawyer
58.1. Subtype: Greedy Lawyer
59.   Role Type: Judge
59.1. Subtype: Immoral Judge
60.   Role Type: Defendant
61.   Role Type: Jury (*see also* Chorus)
62.   Role Type: Witness
63.   Role Type: Prosecutor/Inquisitor

Classification: SOCIOECONOMIC STATUS

64.   Role Type: Lower Class (*see also* Pariah)
65.   Role Type: Working Class/Worker
65.1. Subtype: Brutal Worker
65.2. Subtype: Revolutionary Worker
66.   Role Type: Middle Class
66.1. Subtype: Nouveau Riche
66.2. Subtype: Merchant/Salesperson
66.3. Subtype: Usurer
67.   Role Type: Upper Class
67.1. Subtype: Industrialist/Entrepreneur
67.2. Subtype: Socialite
67.3. Subtype: Servant to the Rich
68.   Role Type: Pariah (*see also* Lost One and Lower Class)
69.   Role Type: Chorus, the Voice of the People

Classification: AUTHORITY AND POWER

70.   Role Type: Warrior
70.1. Subtype: Soldier
70.2. Subtype: Cowardly Soldier (*see also* Braggart Warrior)
70.3. Subtype: Tyrant

71.   Role Type: Police
71.1. Subtype: Clownish Cop
72.   Role Type: Killer
72.1. Subtype: Suicide
72.2. Subtype: Matricide, Parricide, Infanticide, Fratricide

DOMAIN: SPIRITUAL

Classification: NATURAL BEINGS

73.   Role Type: Hero
73.1. Subtype: Superman
73.2. Subtype: Antihero (*see also* Lost One)
73.3. Subtype: Postmodern Antihero
74.   Role Type: Visionary (*see also* Wise Person and Apollonian God/Goddess)
75.   Role Type: Orthodox
75.1. Subtype: Fundamentalist
75.2. Subtype: Ascetic (*see also* Pariah)
76.   Role Type: Agnostic
77.   Role Type: Atheist
77.1. Subtype: Nihilist
78.   Role Type: Cleric
78.1. Subtype: Immoral Cleric
78.2. Subtype: Lapsed Spiritual Leader

Classification: SUPERNATURAL BEINGS

79.   Role Type: God/Goddess
79.1. Subtype: Witty God/Goddess
79.2. Subtype: Dionysian God/Goddess (*see also* Ecstatic One)
79.3. Subtype: Apollonian God/Goddess (*see also* Visionary)
79.4. Subtype: Christ/Saint
80.   Role Type: Fairy (*see also* Fool)
81.   Role Type: Demon (*see also* Beast and Deceiver)
81.1. Subtype: Satan
81.2. Subtype: Death
82.   Role Type: Magician

DOMAIN: AESTHETIC

83.   Role Type: Artist
83.1. Subtype: Performer (*see also* Beauty and Narcissist)
84.   Role Type: Dreamer

References

Aeschylus. (1960 ed.). The Eumenides. In D. Greene & R. Lattimore (Eds.), *Greek Tragedies* (Vol. 3). Chicago: University of Chicago Press.

Allison, R., & Schwarz, T. (1980). *Minds in many pieces*. New York: Rawson, Wade.

Arrowsmith, W. (1970). Introduction. In Aristophanes, *The birds*. New York: New American Library.

Artaud, A. (1958). *The theatre and its double*. New York.: Grove Press.

Axline, V. (1947). *Play therapy*. Boston: Houghton Mifflin.

Beck, J. (1972). *The life of the theatre*. San Francisco: City Lights.

Beckett, S. (1954). *Waiting for Godot*. New York: Grove Press.

Beckett, S. (1968). Come and go. In *Cascando and other short dramatic pieces*. New York: Grove Press.

Berne, E. (1961). *Transactional analysis in psychotherapy*. New York, Grove Press.

Bettelheim, B. (1967). *The empty fortress*. New York: Free Press.

Blake, W. (1960). The tyger. In *Songs of Innocence and of Experience*. New York: Dell. (Original work published 1794)

Blake, W. (1964). Auguries of innocence. In R. Wilbur (Ed.), *Blake*. New York: Dell. (Original work published 1790)

Bloom, B., David, R., & Masia, B. (1956). *Taxonomy of educational objectives: Handbook I: Cognitive domain*. New York: David McKay.

Brissett, D., & Edgley, C. (Eds.). (1975). *Life as theatre: A dramaturgical sourcebook*. Chicago: Aldine.

Brockett, O. (1990). *History of the theatre* (6th ed.). Boston: Allyn & Bacon.

Brook, P. (1978). *The empty space*. New York: Macmillan.

Broucek, F. (1991). *Shame and the self*. New York: Guilford Press.

Bruner, J. S. (1987). The transactional self. In J. S. Bruner & H. Haste (Eds.), *Making sense: The child's construction of the world*. London: Methuen.

Bruner, J. S., & Sherwood, V. (1976). Peekaboo and the learning of rule structures. In J. S. Bruner, A. Jolly, & K. Sylva (Eds), *Play: Its role in development and evolution*. New York: Basic Books.

Buber, M. (1948). *Between man and man*. New York: Macmillan.

Burke, K. (1975). On human behavior considered dramatistically. In D. Brissett & C. Edgley (Eds.), *Life as theatre: A dramaturgical sourcebook*. Chicago: Aldine.

Burns, E. (1972). *Theatricality: A study of convention in the theatre and in social life*. London: Longman.

Byne, W. (1988a). Science and social values: I. A critique of biological theories on the origin of cognitive and behavioral sex differences. *Einstein Quarterly Journal of Biological Medicine, 6,* 58–63.

Byne, W. (1988b). Science and social values: II. A critique of neuroendocrinological theories on the origin of sexual preference. *Einstein Quarterly Journal of Biological Medicine, 6,* 64–70.

Camus, A. (1988). *The stranger.* New York: Knopf. (Original work published 1942)

CBS-TV. (1991, February 27). *48 hours: The many faces of Marsha.*

Chekhov, A. (1935). The marriage proposal. In *The plays of Anton Chekov.* New York: Three Sirens Press.

Conrad, J. (1964). The secret sharer. In *The heart of darkness and the secret sharer.* New York: New American Library. (Original work published 1912)

Cooke, P. (1991, June 23). They cried until the could not see. *New York Times Magazine,* pp. 24–25, 45–48.

Cooley, C. (1922). *Human nature and social order.* New York: Scribner's.

Csikszentmihalyi, M. (1990). *Flow: The psychology of optimal experience.* New York: Harper & Row.

Courtney, R. (1974). *Play, drama and thought.* New York: Drama Book Specialists.

Diderot, D. (1957). *The paradox of acting.* New York: Hill & Wang.

Dostoyevsky, F. (1972). The double. In *Notes from underground and the double.* Baltimore: Penguin Books. (Original work published 1846)

Eliot, T. S. (1963). The love song of J. Alfred Prufrock. In W. R. Benet & N. H. Pearson (Eds.), *The Oxford anthology of American literature.* New York: Oxford University Press. (Original work published 1915)

Emunah, R. (1993). *Acting for real-drama therapy process, technique, and performance.* New York: Brunner/Mazel.

Erikson, E. (1963). *Childhood and society,* New York: Norton.

Federal Bureau of Investigation. (1991). *Statistics.* Washington, DC: Federal Bureau of Investigation.

Fox, J. (Ed.). (1987). *The essential Moreno.* New York: Springer.

Freud, S. (1960). *Totem and taboo.* New York: Random House. (Original work published 1913)

Gassner, J. (1954). *Masters of the drama.* New York: Dover.

Gersie, A. (1991). *Storymaking in bereavement: Dragons fight in the meadows.* London: Kingsley.

Gersie, A., & King, N. (1990). *Storymaking in education and therapy.* London: Kingsley.

Goffman, E. (1959). *The presentation of self in everyday life.* Garden City, NY: Doubleday.

Gould, S. J. (1989). *Wonderful life.* New York: Norton.

Grief, E. (1976). Sex role playing in pre-school children. In J. S. Bruner, A. Jolly, & K. Sylva (Eds.), *Play: Its role in development and evolution.* New York: Basic Books.

Hillman, J. (1983). *Healing fiction.* Tarrytown, NY: Station Hill.

Huizinga, J. (1955). *Homo ludens: A study of the play element in culture.* Boston: Beacon Press.

Irwin, E. (1983). The diagnostic and therapeutic use of pretend play. In C. Shaefer & K. O'Connor (Eds.), *Handbook of play therapy*. New York: Wiley.

Irwin, E. (1985). Puppets in therapy: An assessment procedure. *American Journal of Psychotherapy, 39,* 389–400.

Irwin, E., & Malloy, E. (1975). Family puppet interview. *Family Process, 14,* 179–191.

Irwin, E., & Shapiro, M. (1975). Puppetry as a diagnostic and therapeutic technique. In I. Jakab (Ed.), *Transcultural aspects of psychiatric art* (Vol. 4). Basel: Karger.

James, W. (1950). *The principles of psychology* (Vol. 1). New York: Dover. (Original work published 1890)

Jennings, S. (1990). *The mask, the play, and the paradox: The interface of theatre and therapy.* Keynote address presented at the National Conference of the British Association for Drama Therapy, Newcastle upon Tyne, England.

Jennings, S. (1993). *Theatre, ritual and transformation*. London: Routledge.

Johnson, D. (1981). Drama therapy and the schizophrenic condition. In G. Schattner & R. Courtney (Eds)., *Drama in therapy* (Vol. 2). New York: Drama Book Specialists.

Johnson, D. (1982). Developmental approaches in drama therapy. *The Arts in Psychotherapy, 9,* 183–190.

Johnson, D. (1988). The diagnostic role-playing test. *The Arts in Psychotherapy, 15,* 23–36.

Johnson, D. (1991). The theory and technique of transformations in drama therapy. *The Arts in Psychotherapy, 18,* 285–300.

Jones, E. (1976). *Hamlet and Oedipus*. New York: Norton. (Original work published 1949)

Jung, C. G. (1971). *Psychological types*. Princeton, NJ: Princeton University Press. (Original work published 1921)

Jung, C. G. (1964). *Man and his symbols*. Garden City, NY: Doubleday.

Kafka, F. (1952). A hunger artist. In *Selected short stories of Franz Kafka*. New York: Modern Library. (Original work published 1924)

Kazantzakis, N. (1961). *The last temptation of Christ*. New York: Bantam. (Original work published 1951)

Kirby, E. T. (1975). *Ur-drama: The origins of theatre*. New York: New York University Press.

Klein, M. (1932). *The psychoanalysis of childhood*. London: Hogarth Press.

Kohlberg, L., & Lickona, T. (1986). *The stages of ethical development: From childhood through old age*. San Francisco: Harper San Francisco.

Kritsberg, W. (1988). *The adult children of alcoholics syndrome*. New York: Bantam.

Landy, R. J. (1983). The use of distancing in drama therapy. *The Arts in Psychotherapy, 10,* 175–185.

Landy, R. J. (1986). *Drama therapy: concepts and practices*. Springfield, IL: Charles C Thomas.

Landy, R. J. (1990). The concept of role in drama therapy. *The Arts in Psychotherapy, 17,* 223–230.

Lewis, H. (1971). *Shame and guilt in neurosis*. New York: International Universities Press.

Lichtenstein, T. (1992, April). A mutable mirror: Claude Cahun. *Artforum*, pp. 64–67.

Linton, R. (1936). *The study of man.* New York: Appleton-Century.

Lowenfeld, M. (1979). *The world technique.* London: George Allen & Unwin.

McFarland, B., & Baker-Baumann, T. (1989). *Feeding the empty heart: Adult children of alcoholics and compulsive eating.* San Francisco: Hazelden.

Marmor, J. (1980). *Homosexual behavior: A modern reappraisal.* New York: Basic Books.

Maslow, A. (1962). *Toward a psychology of being.* New York: Van Nostrand Reinhold.

Maslow, A. (1971). *The farther reaches of human nature.* New York: Random House.

Mead, G. H. (1934). *Mind, self and society.* Chicago: University of Chicago Press.

Miller, A. (1981). *The drama of the gifted child.* New York: Basic Books.

Miller, A. (1983). *For your own good.* London: Virago.

Miller, A. (1986). *Thou shalt not be aware: Society's betrayal of the child.* New York: Meridian.

Milton, J. (1957). Paradise lost. In M. Hughes (Ed.), *John Milton: Complete poems and major prose.* New York: Odyssey Press. (Original work published 1667)

Moreno, J. L. (1946). *Psychodrama* (Vol. 1). Beacon, NY: Beacon House.

Moreno, J. L. (1947). *The theatre of spontaneity.* Beacon, NY: Beacon House.

Moreno, J. L. (Ed.). (1960). *The sociometry reader.* Glencoe, IL: Free Press.

National Institute of Mental Health. (1989). *Mental health in the United States.* Washington, DC: U. S. Government Printing Office.

Nietzsche, F. (1956). The birth of tragedy. In *The birth of tragedy and the genealogy of morals.* Garden City, NY: Doubleday. (Original work published 1872)

Noll, R. (1989). Multiple personality, dissociation and C. G. Jung's complex theory. *Journal of Analytical Psychology, 34,* 353–370.

Pearson, C. (1989). *The hero within.* New York: Harper Collins.

Piaget, J. (1926). *The language and thought of the child.* New York: Harcourt, Brace.

Piaget, J. (1965). *Play, dreams and imitation in childhood.* New York: Norton.

Piaget, J., & Inhelder, B. (1969). *The psychology of the child.* New York: Basic Books.

Poe, E. A. (1966). William Wilson. In W. H. Auden (Ed.), *Edgar Allan Poe: Selected prose and poetry.* New York: Holt, Rinehart & Winston. (Original work published 1839)

Portner, E. (1981). *A normative study of the spontaneous puppet stories of eight-year-old children.* Unpublished doctoral dissertation, University of Pittsburgh.

Postman, N. (1984). Social science as theology. *Et Cetera, 41,* 22–33.

Postman, N. (1992). *Technopoly.* New York: Knopf.

Propp, V. (1968). *Morphology of the folktale* (2nd ed.). Austin: University of Texas Press.

Putnam, F. W. (1989). *Diagnosis and treatment of multiple personality disorder.* New York: Guilford Press.

Riso, D. (1987). *Personality types.* Boston: Houghton Mifflin.

Rogers, C. (1961). *On becoming a person.* Boston: Houghton Mifflin.

Roth, P. (1986). *The counterlife.* New York: Farrar Straus, Giroux.

Roth, P. (1993). *Operation Shylock.* New York: Simon & Schuster.

Sacks, O. (1987). *The man who mistook his wife for a hat.* New York: Harper & Row.

Sarbin, T., (1954). Role theory. In G. Lindzey (Ed.), *Handbook of social psychology* (Vol. 1). Reading, MA: Addison-Wesley.

Sarbin, T., (Ed.). (1986). *Narrative psychology.* New York: Praeger.

Sarbin, T., & V. Allen, V. (1968). Role theory. In G. Lindzey & E. Aronson (Eds.), *Handbook of social psychology* (2nd ed., Vol. 1). Reading, MA: Addison-Wesley.

Scheff, T. J. (1979). *Catharsis in healing, ritual and drama.* Berkeley: University of California Press.

Selman, R. L., Lavin, D., & Brion-Meisels, S. (1982). Troubled children's use of self-reflection. In F. Serafica (Ed.), *Social-cognitive development in context.* New York: Guilford Press.

Shakespeare, W. (1959). *Romeo and Juliet.* New York: Washington Square Press. (Original work published 1595)

Shakespeare, W. (1963). *Hamlet.* New York: Washington Square Press. (Original work published 1602)

Shelley, M. (1983). *Frankenstein.* Mattituck, NY: Amerean House. (Original work published 1818)

Sherman, C. (1987). *Cindy Sherman.* New York: Whitney Museum of American Art.

Shipley, J. (1984). *The Crown guide to the world's great plays.* New York: Crown.

Southern, R. (1961). *Seven ages of the theatre.* New York: Hill & Wang.

Stanislavsky, C. (1936). *An actor prepares.* New York: Theatre Arts.

Stevenson, R. L. (1986). *The strange case of Dr. Jekyll and Mr. Hyde.* Chester Springs, PA: Dufour. (Original work published 1886)

Thomas, D. (1957). Do not go gentle into that good night. In *The collected poems of Dylan Thomas.* New York: New Directions.

Tripp, C. A. (1987). *The homosexual matrix.* New York: New American Library.

Turner, V. (1982). *From ritual to theatre.* New York: Performing Arts Journal.

U.S. Bureau of the Census. (1990). *Current population series.* Washington, DC: Department of Commerce.

U.S. Department of Health and Human Services. (1990). *Seventh special report to the United States Congress on alcohol and health.* Washington, DC: U. S. Government Printing Office.

Wilde, O. (1974). *The picture of Dorian Gray.* London: Oxford University Press. (Original work published 1891)

Winnicott, D. W. (1971). *Playing and reality.* London: Tavistock.

Wordsworth, W. (1965). My heart leaps up. In *The prelude, selected poems and sonnets.* New York: Holt, Rinehart & Winston. (Original work published 1807)

Yeats, W. B. (1956). The second coming. In *The collected poems of William Butler Yeats.* New York: Macmillan. (Original work published 1921)

Zamora, M. (1987). *Frida: El pincel de la angustia.* La Herradura, Mexico: Author.

Index